ASSESSING STRESS IN CHILDREN

Louis A. Chandler

PRAEGER

PRAEGER SPECIAL STUDIES • PRAEGER SCIENTIFIC

New York • Philadelphia • Eastbourne, UK
Toronto • Hong Kong • Tokyo • Sydney

Library of Congress Cataloging-in-Publication Data

Chandler, Louis A.
Assessing stress in children.
Bibliography: p.
Includes index.
1. Mental illness – Diagnosis. 2. Stress in children. 3.Child psychopathology. I. Title.
RJ503.5.C46 1985 618.92'89 85-12188
ISBN 0-03-004778-1 (alk. paper)

Published and Distributed by the Praeger Publishers Division (ISBN Prefix 0-275) of Greenwood Press, Inc., Westport, Connecticut

Published in 1985 by Praeger Publishers
CBS Educational and Professional Publishing, a Division of CBS Inc.
521 Fifth Avenue, New York, NY 10175 USA

56789 052 987654321

Printed in the United States of America on acid-free paper

INTERNATIONAL OFFICES

Orders from outside the United States should be sent to the appropriate address listed below. Orders from areas not listed below should be placed through CBS International Publishing, 383 Madison Ave., New York, NY 10175 USA

Australia, New Zealand
Holt Saunders, Pty, Ltd., 9 Waltham St., Artarmon, N.S.W. 2064, Sydney, Australia

Canada
Holt, Rinehart & Winston of Canada, 55 Horner Ave., Toronto, Ontario, Canada M8Z 4X6

Europe, the Middle East, & Africa
Holt Saunders, Ltd., 1 St. Anne's Road, Eastbourne, East Sussex, England BN21 3UN

Japan
Holt Saunders, Ltd., Ichibancho Central Building, 22-1 Ichibancho, 3rd Floor, Chiyodaku, Tokyo, Japan

Hong Kong, Southeast Asia
Holt Saunders Asia, Ltd., 10 Fl, Intercontinental Plaza, 94 Granville Road, Tsim Sha Tsui East, Kowloon, Hong Kong

Manuscript submissions should be sent to the Editorial Director, Praeger Publishers, 521 Fifth Avenue, New York, NY 10175 USA

PREFACE

In recent years there has been considerable pressure for change in mental health practices in our clinics and schools. There are increasing demands for more accountable, economical procedures. Budgetary restraints have forced service providers to be more careful in using limited resources. Critics from within the mental health professions have attacked practices in assessment and intervention on theoretical and methodological grounds. From outside the profession, the pressure for change has come from the civil rights, family privacy, and consumer movements, all of which have contributed to a healthy reexamination of methods and practices.

One response has been a renewed effort to develop more effective and efficient practices of assessment whose validity in decision making can be tested and demonstrated to parents and teachers.

A major impediment to the development of better methods of assessment has been the lack of conceptual agreement among mental health professionals regarding childhood psychopathology. Theoretical differences regarding how to conceptualize the problems of children have retarded the establishment of a widely accepted taxonomy of childhood emotional disorders. Such a taxonomy is essential if progress is to be achieved in the assessment and treatment of children.

This book proposes that professionals who deal with children and their parents adopt a stress paradigm in their theoretical and clinical work. A paradigm which views children with emotional problems in terms of their experience with stress offers several positive features to recommend it.

This can largely be seen as a generic perspective, in the sense that professionals with differing theoretical orientations may find some common ground for agreement within such a broad approach. It can facilitate communication since it has a certain intuitive appeal that recommends such an approach when discussing the problems of children with parents and teachers. It has direct implications for the design, construction, and testing of assessment instruments. And the approach provides a framework for evaluating assessment techniques and methods of treatment.

The method outlined in this book represents an attempt to meet the need for a systematic procedure of assessing, understanding, and helping children.

Louis A. Chandler

TABLE OF CONTENTS

PREFACE v

1 INTRODUCTION 1

Defining the Population 1
The Scope of the Problem 4
The Response of the Schools 6
What Is Needed 28
References 29

2 SOURCES OF STRESS 35

The Study of Stress 35
Stressful Life Events and Situations 40
Special Considerations of Childhood 51
Summary 61
References 61

3 THE EFFECTS OF STRESS 70

Psychophysiological Reactions to Stress 70
Psychological and Behavioral Effects 82
Summary 91
References 91

4 MEDIATORS OF STRESS 99

A Review of the Research 100
Vulnerability to Stress 112
References 119

5 BEHAVIORAL RESPONSES TO STRESS 126

Coping Responses 127
Maladaptive Responses to Stress 130
Summary 143
References 144

6 THE STRESS ASSESSMENT SYSTEM 147

The Children's Life Events Inventory 149
The Need-Threat Scoring System 152
The Stress Response Scale 155
The Structured Parent Interview 158
Clinical Use of the System 160
References 166

7 CHILDREN UNDER STRESS 168

Case Study: Alan T. 168
Case Study: Michael A. 171
Case Study: Brian Z. 172
Case Study: Donny D. 174
Case Study: Judy J. 176
Case Study: Jason E. 177
Case Study: Wilbur T. 179
Case Study: Paul B. 180
Case Study: Robby S. 181

8 INTERVENTION WITH CHILDREN 184

Significant Adults as Agents of Change 185
Methods of Treatment 186
Ronny G.: A Case Study 188
Stress Management Strategies 190
Further Considerations 197
References 199

APPENDIX 205

BIBLIOGRAPHY 225

INDEX 229

ABOUT THE AUTHOR 231

1

INTRODUCTION

All children, in the course of growing up, will experience some of life's inevitable stresses. Such experiences necessitate adjustments which can help the child to develop effective coping resources, and thus foster growth. Excessive and/or prolonged stress however can often have damaging effects. When the child's resources are strained, efforts to cope may not only be ineffective but counterproductive in that they may affect health and impair school performance, as well as relations with parents, other family members, and friends. If the child's efforts to meet the challenge continue to be ineffective, he or she may become frustrated, begin to feel inadequate, and thus develop a poor self image; so the groundwork is laid for more serious emotional problems.

DEFINING THE POPULATION

The focus of this study is children with problems. They are the children who show difficulty in adjusting to the normal demands of growing up in their homes and at school. They may show learning difficulties in school; their performance may be marginal, with occasional failing grades. They are apt to have been retained, or find themselves in remedial classes for reading or math. Some show behavior problems. They may become frustrated with school and get into trouble. Some become shy, reticent, and socially withdrawn; or they may begin to see themselves as bullies, or class clowns. In short, they are not functioning very effectively. Their behavior calls attention to itself, and creates further problems with teachers, parents, and friends.

The children who are the focus of this study are not those with clearly identified intellectual or physical handicaps. For the most part, their condition is not seen as serious enough to qualify for traditional special education programs. They are not mentally retarded, nor do they show clear evidence of the type of neuropsychological deficits associated with the learning disabled, although, in a few of the more severe cases, they may find themselves in special education classes for the emotionally disturbed.

Perhaps these children can best be described as having adjustment problems. If we place such problems on a continuum of severity, theirs might be classified as mild to moderate, as opposed to those so severe as to clearly call for immediate psychological or psychiatric intervention.

Their place on the severity dimension then, provides one parameter for defining this group. They may be further defined by their position on a dimension of duration. For the most part, these children have not shown consistently chronic problems over long periods of time. It is likely that their problems are transient, often situational, reactions. In some cases the problems may be of longer duration, but their manifestations are episodic. A prime characteristic of their behavior is its inconsistency. For a time parents and teachers may report temporary improvement, but further problems emerge often at some later time.

A promising approach to understanding these children can be developed through the study of stress. A stress perspective is immediately suggested by the driven quality of their behavior. These children seem to be responding to some force or stimulus outside of their control, and often outside of their awareness. This stimulus compels them to adopt behavior that is not only ineffective but often counterproductive to their own best interests. We can characterize this stimulus as stress, a state of emotional tension arising from inner needs, life events, or situations. Their extreme behavior then, can be seen as a stress response. Adopting this perspective we can define children with emotional adjustment problems as children who are showing an extreme response to stress.

If stress is the common denominator in cases of children with emotional adjustment problems, then it should be possible to examine the cases of children referred to clinics to identify stressors in their lives. A review of the life histories and current situations of children taken from their clinical reports suggests that stress experiences may be placed in one of three categories: (1) those with overt stressors proximate to the time of referral; (2) those with overt stressors which were not proximate to the time of referral; and (3) those with no obvious overt stressors (what we have called perceived stress situations). The following vignettes illustrate the three types of stress experiences.

The case of Brian provides an illustration of several severe, overt stressors, the experience of which culminated in a referral for clinical services. Brian was a seven-year-old who was having difficulty paying attention in school. He also had begun to show behavior problems, becoming increasingly defiant of authority. An examination of his life history and current situation revealed that his father had died suddenly when he was three years of age. Shortly thereafter his mother was hospitalized for depression. Brian, his brother, and sister, were then placed in a series of foster homes. Midway through Brian's first year in school, the children returned to live with their mother. Brian's learning and behavior problems increased in school so that by the second grade he had been referred for psychological assessment.

By contrast, Donny's case is typical of a child's who has experienced a traumatic event during his early childhood years with lingering effects. Donny was a six-year-old with a history of bedwetting and immature, dependent behavior. He had been having difficulty coping with schoolwork, was receiving poor grades, and was in a special class for reading. An examination of his life history and current situation identified a major event which took place when Donny was two years old. At that time there was a serious fire in the home and, while Donny was not hurt, his younger sister was badly burned. Subsequently, Donny's parents had to spend an inordinate amount of time with his sister, taking her for frequent treatments to the burn clinic. Although Donny seemed initially to cope well with that trauma, he showed increasing problems once he started kindergarten, and in first grade he was referred for psychological services.

Finally, Judy's case was one where no overt stressors were evident, but she was responding as though she were under stress. This was seen as a case of perceived stress situations. Judy was a seven-year-old whose behavior was concerning her parents and teachers because of her frequent demands for attention and approval. She showed a strong need to be liked and sought affection from adults and peers at every possible opportunity. An examination of her life situation and history showed no overt stressors; however, a subsequent personality assessment found that Judy saw the world as a place in which she had been deprived of love. Her strong needs for affiliation and fears of rejection created stress for her in interpersonal situations, and she responded with the driven quality of children under stress.

THE SCOPE OF THE PROBLEM

Estimates of the number of children in need of mental health services vary widely. Prevalence rates are difficult to establish because of the lack of clear, agreed-upon definitions for mental disorders. Differences in theoretical viewpoints, terminology, professional orientation, and research methodology all contribute to the confusion. Nevertheless, some general estimates of the scope of the problem can be made.

Surveys of relatively large populations of normal children shed some light on the matter. Lapouse and Monk (1958, 1959) used mothers' responses to a structured interview to examine 482 normal children, ages six to 12 years. They found relatively high percentages had symptoms which were often associated with adjustment problems. For example, 43 percent had seven or more current fears and worries. Werry and Quay (1971) surveyed all the children in kindergarten through second grade in Urbana, Illinois. Using teacher ratings, they reported that 46 percent of the boys were rated as disruptive; 23 percent as showing odd, bizarre behavior; 43 percent as having a short attention span; and so forth.

A more recent report, prepared by the New York State Department of Mental Hygiene (1974), concluded that approximately 4 to 5 percent of the children in an elementary school population would be perceived by teachers as having persistent emotional problems. Of particular interest to the current study are the estimates prepared by Clarizio and McCoy (1978). They estimated that approximately one in every ten public school children has a moderate to severe adjustment problem. They went on to say that if those with mild adjustment problems were included, the ratio would increase to about three out of ten.

Because of the relatively low level of severity and the episodic quality of behavior, it is likely that many of these children are never formally identified as in need of services. As a result, they are probably underrepresented in statistical data.

Still other evidence that suggests the scope of the problem comes from the study of rapid social changes and the resulting pressures placed on the family. Life changes, such as divorce, unconventional living arrangements, the changing roles of women, parental job loss, and family moves and relocations, contribute to instability in the child's environment and disruption in the family, thus having a direct impact on children.

Of these various changes, the incidence of divorce is probably the best documented. The divorce ratio has more than doubled from 1970 to 1981, and more than tripled since 1960 (Guidubaldi, 1983). Today, one out of five children in the average classroom lives in a single-parent home (Drake and Shellenberger, 1981). Hetherington (1979) estimates that 40 to 50 percent of the children born in the past decade will spend some time living in a single-parent family. Since 75 percent of all divorces occur in families with children under 18 years of age, and since it is estimated that 40 percent of the current marriages of young adults will end in divorce (Glick and Norton, 1978), it becomes apparent that growing numbers of children will have to cope with the impact of divorce.

Crisis events such as divorce and separation can cause marked changes in children's behavior, particularly in school (Drake and Shellenberger, 1981). There is also evidence to suggest that children of divorce are likely to show aggressive, acting-out behavior (McDermott, 1970; Kalter, 1977). Increased restlessness, obstinacy, disruptiveness, and impulsiveness are among the other behaviors frequently reported (Felner, Stolberg, and Cowen, 1975). Children's emotional reactions have been found to include confusion, anger, guilt, fear, and depression (Kelly and Wallerstein, 1977).

THE RESPONSE OF THE SCHOOLS

Among the first groups of children to be identified as needing some sort of special education procedures were the mentally retarded. Modern efforts to provide such services can be traced to nineteenth-century France. Education in republican France remained under the influence of the Enlightenment, with its emphasis on humanistic principles. As steps were taken to widen the availability of secular education to increasing numbers of children, it became apparent that some were so limited that they could not keep up with their classmates. They learned at a slower rate, and seemed much more limited in their capabilities.

In the fall of 1904 the Ministry of Public Instruction in Paris sought the advice of the noted psychologist Alfred Binet for a means of identifying these slow learners. As a solution to this problem, Binet designed a series of structured sequential tasks, a test that could be used to identify children who were mentally deficient and thus in need of special education. In time special education and training programs were developed for the mentally retarded and the idea that some groups of children, because of their unique problems or handicapping conditions, might need special education began to grow.

Special Education for the Emotionally Disturbed

Special education was developed for children with vision and hearing problems, and for the physically handicapped. In more recent times, children with psychoneurological learning disabilities were seen as a group that would need special education programing. Such categorical service delivery assumed that children could be grouped into, more or less, homogeneous groups, based on some primary handicapping condition that they all shared. Special programs could then be tailored based on the psychological and educational understanding of the handicapping condition. Following this categorical approach, it seemed logical to provide special classes for children who were emotionally disturbed.

The first attempts to provide special education for emotionally disturbed children had probably been those which came about when hospitals and institutions began to introduce educational programs for their children patients. In one such pioneering attempt, Dr. Lauretta Bender organized the children's ward at the Bellevue Psychiatric Hospital in New York City, and in 1934 asked the Board of Education to provide teachers to staff the classrooms. During the next two decades education became an increasingly important component in residential treatment and other institutions for psychiatric care. For the most part, these classes were designed for inpatients, and so dealt with children whose conditions were so serious that they required hospitalization or institutionalization.

In 1946 the New York City Board of Education organized special public schools to educate emotionally disturbed and maladjusted children. Private schools, specifically founded to serve that population, also began to gain prominence at this time. Gradually throughout the 1950s the public schools began to take an increasing responsibility for educating children with emotional problems.

During the 1960s special education classes for the emotionally disturbed proliferated (Barack, 1984). It was also during the 1960s that the federal government began to take a wider role. In 1963 Public Law 88-164 provided federal support for the preparation of personnel to work with disturbed children. Much of the thrust provided by the federal initiative culminated, in 1978, in the passage of Public Law 94-142, which affirmed the right of all handicapped children to a free and appropriate public education. One effect of this law was to increase the opportunities available for the emotionally disturbed within the educational mainstream, since such children could no longer be excluded from public school programs because of their handicapping conditions.

As educational programs evolved, the limits of the categorical approach to special education became apparent. This was especially the case in dealing with the emotionally disturbed. When special services for institutionalized children were extended to children in the regular public schools, the nature and severity of the problems began to change. Schizophrenic children and those with school refusal problems could be categorized together as "emotionally disturbed." Moreover, since some criteria had to be adopted for making decisions regarding group membership (necessitated by this approach), many children were excluded from help because their condition was not, at the time of the assessment, seen as severe enough to qualify them for special education placement. Even with the best of efforts the criteria for entrance into those programs often seemed vague, relying principally on psychiatric judgment and the opinions of psychologists and teachers as to whether the child's emotional state constituted a condition so severe as to significantly impair school functioning.

This approach tended to limit services to relatively small numbers of children with severe emotional disorders, or those whose behavior had become so disruptive that they were difficult to deal with in the regular education classes.

Once a child had qualified for special services, the services actually available might vary considerably. Programmatically, such service would include a teacher who had had some specialized training, placement in a classroom of limited enrollment--which might allow a closer monitoring of individual learning and behavior--and occasional psychiatric or psychological consultation available to the teacher. Extended services, such as child psychotherapy or family counseling, have not usually been provided by the schools, although a local mental health agency might have some responsibilities in those areas.

The Categorical Approach to Special Education

Even as the limits of the categorical approach were becoming increasingly evident, another factor served to blur the distinction between those identified as emotionally maladjusted and their "normal" peers: that was the mainstreaming movement in special education.

Mainstreaming is a term that has been used to describe the efforts to meet the special needs of children in conditions approaching the normal classroom environment. It is based on a conceptual view of special education as a continuum of instructional arrangements ranging from the more restrictive ones, like specialized residential schools, to less restrictive ones, like the regular class (Reynolds and Birch, 1977). The guiding principle is that children should be given an appropriate education within the least restrictive environment, a principle given legal sanction in Public Law 94-142.

It became possible, applying the mainstreaming principle, for an emotionally maladjusted child to be seated in a regular classroom next to a "normal" child, who might be showing emotional adjustment difficulties. Clearly, the categorical distinctions seemed to lose some validity with this sort of arrangement. It seemed more useful to conceptualize emotional adjustment problems on a continuum of severity.

Still another aspect of the categorical approach which came under considerable criticism was the labeling that was a necessary part of group identification. Since the scientific study of child psychopathology requires some conceptual relationships, classification and the naming of categories are a necessary function. Unfortunately, such clinical terms are often misinterpreted by the public; they may carry socially undesirable connotations; and in some cases, they may take on a social stigma.

Johns and Johns (1982) give an excellent illustration of one result of the labeling problem in special education in discussing the phenomenal growth in the number of children labeled as learning disabled (LD). They point out that that label is one of the least offensive to parents and professional groups, and so efforts are made to have children who are having problems in school labeled as LD, so that they may be eligible to receive special education services. The result has been that the total population of students labeled as LD doubled in the 1970s and is still increasing.

Given the development of special education services, it seems evident that many children who might need help in their emotional adjustment will find no systematic means for getting that help in the schools. The final factor which limits the help available is the diminishing of special education resources. There has been a recent reexamination of financial resources in education. Cutbacks and layoffs have become common in the nation's school systems. There are increased demands to do more with less. There are also legitimate demands being made for more efficient and effective programs in the schools. A concomitant demand for practices that lend themselves to evaluation has grown as schools and teachers are being held more accountable by the public for the quality of educational programs.

A Typical School's Response: The Rogers School Study

In 1978 the University of Pittsburgh and the Pittsburgh Board of Public Education engaged in a joint project to provide psychological services to a selected school. A major aim of this project was to develop and demonstrate alternative ways of organizing school psychological services.

The traditional role of the school psychologist had evolved along with the categorical approach to special education. In this role the school psychologist acted as a gatekeeper to special education programs. Typically, children were referred to the psychologist with a wide variety of learning and behavior problems. A battery of psychoeducational tests were then administered to the child, and the results placed against the criteria for entrance into special education. Within this paradigm, the child either qualified or not for one of the various programs. The school psychologist's recommendation included the results of this yes/no decision.

This process was labor-intensive, and because of professional time constraints, only relatively small numbers of children could be seen by the school psychologist. Moreover, by forcing the issue into a discrete yes/no outcome, the implication remained that, short of special education placement, there was relatively little the school could offer.

The James C. Rogers School was an urban elementary school located near the university. It had a school population of 340 children in grades kindergarten through eight. The psychological services available to the school were typical of those provided throughout the city, and similar to the arrangements commonly found throughout the country. A school psychologist was assigned by the district to Rogers School, two other elementary schools, and one middle school. Because of the scheduling requirements of several locations and a considerable workload, professional time was spent conducting psychological assessments with those children whose problems had become so severe that they were being seen on a "crisis" or priority basis. An examination of school records showed that, for one three-semester period, 88 children had been referred for diagnostic psychological assessment.

The demonstration project provided faculty and doctoral students as psychoeducational consultants for teachers and administrators. A lower level, less intensive, case review procedure was inserted into the referral process by having the teacher refer children to the school psychologist through a field-training clinic established in the school.

After cases had been filtered through the clinic, those most clearly in need of a comprehensive psychological assessment were passed on to the school psychologist.

The results showed that there was a dramatic decline in the number of children referred for psychological assessment when alternative methods were offered to teachers. There was a total of 38 assessments completed during the three-semester life of the project, comparable to the baseline period (when 88 had been completed). Moreover, during this time 91 children were referred to the training clinic staff, suggesting that teachers were eager and willing to call upon the staff in this consulting capacity when the service was made available to them.

The experience at Rogers School illustrates the practical limits of the categorical approach and points to the need for lower level interventions for larger numbers of children. It shows that children with problems can be seen on a continuum of severity, and that a continuum of interventions can be designed to meet their needs. Such efforts made earlier in the referral process might allow some problems to be effectively dealt with so that they not develop into more serious problems demanding more intensive intervention at some later time. In this sense, early low-level intervention is preventive.

The Response of the Mental Health Professions

The treatment of the emotional problems of children, like the study of child psychopathology itself, has evolved from the study of adult mental disorders. For much of the history of the mental health movement, the problems of children were not directly addressed. The earliest clinic for children was founded in 1896 by Lightner Witmer at the University of Pennsylvania. Witmer advocated employing educational methods to help children with school problems. In 1912 a psychoeducational clinic was established at the University of Pittsburgh for "the accurate diagnosis of educationally and mentally unusual children . . ." (Boyd, 1977).

There were other isolated examples of efforts specifically to address the problems of children, but it remained for the mental hygiene movement to promote widespread attention to the treatment of children's disorders.

That movement had developed from the principles outlined by Clifford Beers in his book, A Mind That Found Itself, published in 1907. His ideas were, in turn, influenced by such early American pioneers as William James and Adolf Meyer. For Beers, prevention was fundamental to mental health practices. His book, with its blueprint for reforming mental hospitals, was instrumental in launching the mental hygiene movement. In 1909 the National Committee for Mental Hygiene was organized, with Beers as its executive secretary.

The movement was to have a considerable influence on the development of mental health services in the United States. It was instrumental in advocating specialized training programs for psychiatric social workers. It also turned public attention to the problems of school children.

In 1915 the National Committee surveyed the existing services for children and found them woefully lacking. During the following years, the Committee developed programs and demonstration projects that created a movement for child guidance clinics. The growth of such clinics was further fostered by the establishment, in 1924, of the American Orthopsychiatric Association, an interdisciplinary organization of mental health professionals which works with children and their families.

The child guidance clinic has become one of the more important focal points for the treatment of children with emotional disorders. Such clinics are generally organized around a model of service delivery that includes interviews with the parents, psychological testing with the child, and follow-up treatment consisting of child psychotherapy, family counseling, parent guidance, or some combination of treatments. Generally, the clinics are staffed by social workers, psychologists, and psychiatrists, each providing some portion of the service. This child guidance model has influenced treatment programs in a variety of settings, such as community mental health agencies, hospitals, and residential treatment facilities for children.

The Classification of Children's Disorders

The child guidance model recognized the importance of an accurate assessment of the problem. Information gathered by parent interview, psychological testing of the child, and psychiatric examination all contribute to an assessment of the nature and severity of the problem. Effective intervention can best be planned from the understanding of the child derived from a comprehensive assessment.

Psychological assessment is a process of sequential decision making the objective of which is the understanding and prediction of behavior. It is a scientific inquiry employing analytic, deductive reasoning. The process, in the case of clinical assessment, can be seen as an inquiry into the nature and severity of the referring problem. The inquiry proceeds along a series of decision points, each requiring a formulation of alternatives, evaluation among the alternatives, and a single solution which leads to the next decision point. These decision points may be framed as a series of diagnostic questions.

Identification of the appropriate questions requires some familiarity with the concepts in the field of study and their relationships within the general domain. In this case the field of study is child psychopathology, and the possible alternatives would be found in a taxonomy of children's emotional disorders. If the ultimate aim of psychological assessment is prediction, the key role of an adequate diagnostic classification system becomes evident. Prediction is based on a knowledge of how similar subjects behaved in similar situations; and individual predictions can only be made, in terms of probability, when placed against data from a larger sample. The similarities of subjects allows them to be grouped according to some schema and, from that classification, predictions can be made. The need for an adequate taxonomy is crucial in refining predictions and advancing the science. In order to understand the problems associated with establishing a taxonomy, a brief historical digression might be useful.

For much of its history the study of child psychopathology was seen as a footnote to adult psychopathology. Diagnostic assessment, classification, and treatment techniques were often those used with adults, with minor modifications made to adapt them for children. In order to understand the development of classification systems for children's disorders, it is necessary to know something of the history of classification of adult mental disorders.

The scientific study of mental disorder is a relatively recent human endeavor. For centuries the mentally ill were considered as society's outcasts. Their problems were, at various times in history, attributed to vile body fluids, noxious ethers, witchcraft, demonic possession, or mental deficiency. Depending on their society's point of view, their "treatment" might consist of bloodletting, exorcism, public humiliation, social isolation, or burning at the stake.

A movement for a more humane treatment was begun in the wake of the French Enlightenment, in the eighteenth century. Phillipe Pinel (1745-1826), a pioneer in the reform movement, obtained permission from the French authorities to release mental patients from their chains and introduce a more humanitarian treatment consisting of fresh air, exercise, and work. Gradually, as the specialty of psychiatry came into its own, mental disorders began to be seen as illness requiring medical treatment.

While the humanistic principles of the Enlightenment were to influence the care of the mentally ill, it was the scientific principles that revolutionized the study of mental disorders. By common agreement, modern science dates its birth from the publication of Copernicus' epoch work on astronomy in 1543. In 1637, Descartes published his Discourse on Method in which he paved the way for the application of mathematical methods to the investigation of scientific problems. In the hundred years between the two events, a number of major works were published in the physical sciences. Gilbert's De Magnete, usually credited as one of the first, was published in 1600. Dated from this epoch, the history of modern science spans about 400 years.

By the sixteenth and seventeenth centuries, physics, anatomy, chemistry, and biology were revolutionized by the adoption of systematic methods of inquiry. The new approach was analytic, and it was empirical--based on experience. It held that natural phenomena could be objectively observed, measured, classified, and categorized, and thus understood; and from that understanding predictions could be made.

Classification and categorization were integral elements of the new method which facilitated the organization of knowledge. These features of the scientific method were best exemplified in the work of the Swedish botanist, Carolus Linnaeus. Linnaeus was to spend much of his career developing a nomenclature and system of classification for the study of plants and animals. He found a muddled, confused, chaotic situation where workers could find little agreement among themselves. His great task was to bring some order out of that chaos. Arthur O. Lovejoy described his contribution this way:

> He was an unsurpassed organizer . . . he introduced form and order, clearness and precision, simple definitions and plain delimitations of boundaries into sciences more or less chaotic or confused or impeded with cumbrous and inappropriate categories and terminology (Downs, 1961).

The increasing acceptance of scientific methods in medicine and psychology brought into focus the need for a taxonomy of mental disorders. Like the situation Linnaeus had found in biology some 150 years earlier, psychiatric practices in the nineteenth century tended to be idiosyncratic with little communication among practitioners and researchers, mainly because of the lack of an agreed-upon set of definitions. Diagnosis was often confused and contradictory. Treatment was tentative and difficult to evaluate. It became apparent that the lack of an adequate taxonomy was impeding progress.

One of the first pioneers to attempt to deal with the problem was Emil Kraepelin (1856-1926). Kraepelin was a German psychiatrist who devoted much of his professional career to the task of classifying mental disorders. He reasoned that, like the physical ailments, mental diseases could be classified by onset, symptom development, and outcomes. Kraepelin's work, and especially his contributions on dementia praecox and manic-depressive psychosis, was to have a considerable influence on modern psychiatry. His descriptive classification schemes, modified and revised, were to become the basis for the first edition of the American Psychiatric Association's official taxonomy, as presented in their Diagnostics and Statistical Manual of Mental Disorders (DSM-I) in 1952.

As workers began to adopt the DSM categories, a number of inadequacies became apparent. This was especially true in its treatment of children's disorders. In order to correct these weaknesses, a number of competing taxonomies were proposed, so that by 1966 the Group for the Advancement of Psychiatry, in reviewing the classification of childhood psychopathology, concluded that more than 20 different systems had been proposed.

By the 1960s advances in the understanding of emotional disorders necessitated the first revision of the DSM. It was also in the early 1960s that the development of more powerful statistical techniques for psychological applications began to influence research by providing new tools for identifying and validating clinical syndromes. Techniques such as cluster analysis and factor analysis allowed the researcher to examine the interrelationships among disparate elements. Using such means, it became possible to identify symptoms that seemed likely to be found together. One of the earliest studies using these techniques with children's behavior problems was reported by Peterson in 1961. By examining symptom clusters in a population of school children with behavioral disturbance, Peterson was able to identify two factors as relatively stable over time. He labeled these conduct problems and personality problems.

Jenkins (1966) used a cluster analysis technique on a 90-symptom checklist to classify 500 cases of behavior disorders of children and adolescents. He found five symptomatic clusters: shy-seclusive, overanxious, hyperactive, undomesticated, and socialized delinquent. He grouped these subtypes into two types which he labeled as inhibited and aggressive. These five clusters were to constitute the basis for the classification of behavior disorders found in the second edition of the DSM (DSM-II, 1968) (Mezzich, 1979).

The attempt was also made, in the second edition, to develop a descriptive approach. This was an approach that would be, as much as possible, atheoretical in terms of etiology and process. Continuing progress and experience gained with the DSM-II led to another revision begun in the mid-1970s and published in 1980, the DSM-III.

The new edition sought to recognize the complexity of mental problems by incorporating a multiaxial diagnostic system. Diagnosis on Axes I and II were to include the mental disorders. Axis III was reserved for physical disorders and conditions; Axis IV for the severity of psychosocial stressors; Axis V for an estimate of the highest level of adaptive functioning during the past year. Other important changes were made in the classification of children's disorders. A new designation label for disorders that are first evident in infancy, childhood, or adolescence was proposed. Children might be assigned a diagnosis from among this group, or they might be assigned another diagnosis from among the adult groups. There were four times as many categories in this new section as there were in the childhood sections of DSM-II, reflecting a considerable increase in knowledge in that area (Spitzer, Williams, and Skodol, 1980). The diagnoses in this class were divided into five major groups based on the predominant area of disturbance: intellectual, behavioral, emotional, physical, and developmental. Table 1.1 outlines the major diagnostic categories in each area. DSM-III also maintained the atheoretical stance by providing descriptive statements and diagnostic criteria, but generally avoiding statements regarding etiology.

TABLE 1.1

Major Disorders Usually First Evident in Infancy, Childhood, or Adolescence

Intellectual
Mental retardation
Behavioral/Emotional
Attention deficit disorder
Conduct disorder
Anxiety disorder
Other disorders of infancy, childhood, or adolescence
Physical
Eating disorders
Stereotypic movement disorders
Other disorders with physical manifestations
Developmental
Pervasive developmental disorders
Specific developmental disorders

While the descriptive approach continued to be developed in the DSM-III, efforts were also continuing to identify disorders by empirical methods. Quay (1972), in reviewing many statistical studies, concluded that three patterns consistently emerged, although investigators used a variety of labels. He subsumed the various factors under the labels of aggressive, withdrawn, and immature. (He also identified a fourth factor which was unlike the others since it was seen as a response to environmental conditions. This he labeled socialized delinquent.)

More recently, there have been several promising attempts to develop data-based classifications of children's disorders (Achenbach and Edelbrock, 1978; Dreger, 1977; Mezzich, 1979; Edelbrock, 1979; Quay, 1983). Edelbrock (1979), in reviewing the efforts in empirical classification of children's behavior disorders, pointed out that while there had been a number of screening instruments developed to identify disturbed children, few differentiated among disturbed children. That is, few instruments were capable of allowing classification into subtypes. After reviewing a number of instruments, he concluded that there was considerable evidence for the existence of two broad band syndromes: overcontrolled and undercontrolled. He found less evidence for the existence of a broad band syndrome characterizing learning problems, and he further maintained that a fourth band characterizing immature behavior had only been identified in studies using Peterson's Problem Checklist.

Edelbrock concluded that there had been few efforts to translate empirically derived syndromes into categories, due in part to the lack of an established diagnostic system against which empirically derived syndromes could be validated.

As has been pointed out, meaningful psychological assessment is dependent upon an adequate taxonomy. Edelbrock has implied that it is also possible to proceed inductively, that is, to derive a taxonomy based on data gathered by assessment instruments. In order to better understand the relationship between classification and assessment, it may be useful to review the historical development of psychological assessment.

A Historical Review of Psychological Assessment

Scientific psychology is generally dated from the founding of the first psychological laboratory by Wilhelm Wundt in 1879. Wundt was influential in defining the methods and content of the new psychology. The methods used would be those of experimental science. By identifying the problems he would study, he gradually furthered the process of separating psychology from philosophy and physiology. According to Wundt, psychological studies should investigate sensations and feelings, thoughts, volitions, perceptions, and emotions. This was the proper content of psychological study. In order to investigate these phenomena, Wundt applied the scientific methods of careful observation and measurement to the performance of his human subjects.

The period from 1890 to 1905 has been called the "laboratory" period in mental measurements (Sattler, 1982). During this period tests were invented for measuring individual responses in the laboratories, and these tests gradually found application in the practice of psychology. From this early work, the methods, applications, and techniques were developed for the study of individual differences.

It was during this period that Francis Galton, working in England, furthered the study of individual differences by developing statistical techniques for describing the characteristics he measured on various laboratory tasks. In 1882 Galton founded a laboratory where human subjects were asked to take a series of tests measuring such physical characteristics as reaction time and sensory functioning. These formally structured tasks were the first attempts at modern mental tests. While Galton had developed methods and apparatus for psychological measurement, what gave his work particular importance were the statistical techniques that made it possible to express the results in quantitative terms. He applied the normal probability curve to his laboratory measurements as a way of understanding human variability. In the process he demonstrated that many physical and psychological characteristics were distributed according to a bell-shaped curve.

James McKeen Cattell was an American student of Wundt's who was influenced by Galton's work. He pursued the study of individual differences, measuring a number of responses including attention span, sensory functioning, and motor and perceptual skills. Cattell is credited with first introducing the term "mental test." Galton and Cattell's work set the direction for the development of mental testing by introducing many of the techniques and methods that are still in use today.

Toward the turn of the century, the newly established field of psychometrics was to take a significant step forward with the work of Alfred Binet. Binet, like Galton, believed that the basic concept for individual psychology should focus upon deviations from a population average (Linden and Linden, 1968). He proceeded to find, by experimentation, what tasks a child might be expected to perform at a given age. By trial and error, with hundreds of tasks given to large numbers of children, he was able eventually to come up with 54 tasks which could be arranged by degree of difficulty according to age expectancies. A child's mental age could then be computed by his performance on this set of tasks. If his overall performance was significantly below that of the average child of his age, he might be identified as needing special educational help. Binet had designed a test which was able to distinguish between normal and retarded children.

The tasks Binet developed, in collaboration with Theophile Simon, would eventually be used in the construction of the first intelligence test. The Stanford-Binet Intelligence Scale, a revision of Binet's original scale by Lewis Terman, was to be for many years the most widely used intelligence test in the United States and in many other countries.

Binet's scale represented one of the true success stories of psychometrics, and although it has become fashionable in recent years to criticize intelligence tests on various social grounds, the intelligence test stands as a singular achievement in psychological testing. Cronbach (1970) has called it the most important technical contribution psychology has made to the practical guidance of human affairs.

Binet's effort is instructive for another reason. It illustrated the inductive approach to problem solving. Binet did not set out with a grand theory of intelligence. He did not, at first, seek to define it. Rather, he built his scale by amassing hundreds of single observations of children for the practical reason of developing an instrument which could distinguish between two groups. Only as his work proceeded was some effort made to clarify the concept of intelligence.

Scientific reasoning employs two major forms of logic, the deductive and the inductive. Deductive reasoning is from the general to the specific, from a general scientific principle to the occurrence of the particular event in accordance with that principle. Deductive logic relies on theory to provide the general statement. Inductive logic is reasoning which proceeds from the specific to the general where principles are derived from observations of numerous specific instances. Binet's approach was inductive, relying as he did on many observations of children's responses to test items. The distinction is an important one in test construction.

Many early psychological tests were based on current psychological theories. The authors derived, from some theoretical perspective, those test items that seemed logically to represent the condition or dimension being studied. These items were then arranged in a test format.

Lanyon and Goodstein (1982) refer to this as the theoretical-rational approach to test construction. The Woodworth Personal Data Sheet, for example, was an early rating scale, developed during World War I, which, in the opinion of those constructing the test, contained items indicative of "neuroticism." A later development, the Bernreuter Personality Inventory (1931), is more typical of this period. This test consisted of 125 items that yielded six scores in the areas of neurotic tendency, self-sufficiency, introversion-extraversion, dominance-submission, sociability, and self-confidence. Some instruments were more explicitly grounded in a specific theoretical position. Instruments such as the Allport-Vernon-Lindzey Study of Values and the Edwards Personal Preference Schedule were carefully constructed in accordance with contemporary personality theory.

While early researchers were struggling with the problems of quantifying psychological data, a different approach began to emerge, given impetus by the psychoanalytic principles of Sigmund Freud, and exemplified by the technique of Hermann Rorschach. Rorschach's psychodiagnostic technique, described in his 1921 book, was designed as a method for the appraisal of personality. Rorschach experimented with hundreds of inkblots, eventually settling on a set of ten plates which were to become the standard set. The plates were presented sequentially to the subject who was encouraged to provide associations and interpretations. There was no attempt to impose structure or limit the responses. Instead the subject was allowed to generate his unique response pattern. The significance of various aspects of the response could only be judged in terms of the individual's total response pattern.

L. K. Frank (1939) was later to coin the term "projective technique" for such methods which employed a relatively unstructured stimulus given meaning by the subject. This approach to the study of personality, focusing as it did on individual responses, made few attempts to group data or compare responses among individuals. Unlike psychometric tests, these techniques did not lend themselves well to quantitative interpretation and statistical treatment.

The first half of the twentieth century saw psychology evolve from a laboratory science to an applied science, and the major area of application was in psychological testing. Clinical psychology arose as practitioners were trained to administer intelligence tests and later to perform diagnostic assessments using the newly developed projective techniques. The clinical psychologist became a psychodiagnostician whose expanding role in mental health services was concerned with the assessment of the patient's emotional condition.

This emphasis on psychodiagnostics, in turn, led to increased reliance on projective techniques. Rorschach's technique was followed by Henry Murray's Thematic Apperception Test. Murray had introduced the new technique in an article published in 1935 (Morgan and Murray, 1935). His test consisted of a set of pictures designed to elicit stories from the subject. Drawing heavily on psychoanalytic principles, Murray suggested that the stories subjects produced represented the inner dynamics of personality. The method was based on the supposition that when someone is asked to interpret a complex social situation, he is apt to tell us as much about himself as he is about the situation on which his attention is focused.

This line of work encouraged others and a number of techniques were spawned seeking to analyze responses to various stimuli. But even as projective techniques proliferated and found widespread use with the growth of clinical psychology in the 1930s and 1940s, criticisms were growing. Critics complained that the projective approach to personality assessment, relying as it did on the individual's unique response and the idiosyncratic meaning which he gave to the stimuli, did not lend itself well to scientific study, testing, and validation.

By the 1950s, questions of validity and reliability could no longer be ignored. Paul Meehl's (1954) highly influential monograph did much to clarify the issue. Meehl set out to analyze the process of clinical prediction. While the process the clinician used in arriving at a diagnosis was often private and inaccessible, he reasoned that it should be capable of being subjected to the same sort of empirical standards that were applied to statistical prediction. Meehl went on to review the empirical studies which had attempted to compare clinical and statistical prediction methods.

After examining the few available studies, he concluded that the overwhelming weight of the evidence showed the superiority of statistical over traditional clinical methods. Meehl's findings sparked considerable controversy and clearly framed an important issue for the clinical assessment of personality.

The statistical methods which Meehl had found to be superior were the result of advances in psychometrics. Such efforts were typified by the work of a group of researchers at the University of Minnesota, which resulted in the development, in the late 1930s, of the Minnesota Multiphasic Personality Inventory (MMPI). This instrument was designed for routine diagnostic assessment. One of the test's authors described the impetus for the test this way:

> It was the sheer frustration of the need for a more practical if not more valid test to use in clinical applications of psychology which led to the development of the first thoroughly empirical personality inventory (Hathaway, 1965).

It was hoped then that a group-administered inventory could provide a more efficient method for routine psychodiagnostic evaluation. In many ways, the inventory was a departure from traditional test construction. The authors, in constructing the MMPI, employed an empirical item-selection procedure based on different response frequencies between normal and clinical groups. Such inventories are described as criterion-keyed because they are composed of items that significantly differentiate between two or more criterion groups (Aiken, 1976).

The MMPI was an empirically validated structured test. It was an objective (rather than projective) test. As such, data could be grouped and test performance compared. It was an instrument which, in turn, lent itself to empirically derived rules for making clinical decisions. Such rules could be provided to the examiner as a set of "cookbook" procedures. Meehl presented arguments to show that for given psychometric patterns, personality descriptions could be generated by such automatic, mechanical, clerical "cookbook" procedures (Meehl, 1956; Marks and Seeman, 1963). With this approach, individuals were grouped into test-determined classes (Gilberstadt and Duker, 1965). This differed from the more traditional approach to test construction which relied more on the face or content validity of items to establish their membership in various classes.

It became increasingly obvious, however, as researchers and clinicians worked with the MMPI that in at least one major sense it failed to live up to expectations.

ment gives rise to a host of possible interpretations and technical questions about test validity (see Jensen, 1981, for a more thorough discussion of this issue).

Personality Assessment

In addition to the criticisms leveled at the use of various ability and aptitude tests in employment, the use of personality tests was singled out for especially harsh censure. By 1965, the criticisms of testing and social research had become so vocal that congressional hearings on the subject were held (Amrine, 1965; Lovell, 1967). The practice of requiring applicants to take personality tests was closely examined (Aiken, 1976).

Perhaps because of their clinical applications and the public's perception of them, personality tests are an emotionally laden subject. The notion that these tests are a kind of psychic x-ray laying bare one's inner secrets lends this type of testing a mystique which understandably raises fears. A knowledge of a candidate's personality characteristics for personnel, military, or student selection procedures might be useful, but that must be balanced against the danger of invasion of privacy. This danger is lessened only a little by the assurance that the candidate's participation in the process is "voluntary."

Cronbach (1970) makes an interesting ethical distinction between personality testing conducted for institutions and that conducted for an individual. In the first instance, tests are given to meet specific institutional objectives; in the second, they serve to benefit the individual. As Cronbach has pointed out, any test is an invasion of privacy for the subject who does not wish to reveal himself.

Intellectual Assessment

The use of the IQ test has been called one of the burning issues in psychology today (Clarizio, 1979). Mental tests, and particularly IQ tests, have a long history in the schools. It might be remembered that Binet's original test was developed for use in educational decision making. The similar use of tests today has become an especially controversial issue as when they are utilized to make decisions on educational placement (for example, whether or not a child should be considered mentally retarded).

The recent criticisms of testing in the schools might be traced back to the Supreme Court decision in Brown v. Board of Education (1954) which held that the public schools must be desegregated. Civil rights advocates saw educational and psychological tests as tools being used to hinder integration. Subsequently, there was an explosion of legislation and litigation affecting psychological testing (Bersoff, 1980). The storm of criticism broke when it was found that a disproportionately large number of minority children had been placed in classes for slow learners or the retarded in several communities. This became the issue behind a number of very important court decisions (Hobsen vs. Hansen [1967]; P. v. Riles [1972]; Diana v. California State Board of Education [1970]). Critics saw it as prima facie evidence that the tests were biased against minority groups.

In the early 1970s, a number of legislative initiatives reflected the growing concern. In 1972, a bill was introduced in the California State Legislature which would have abolished statewide testing of IQ or scholastic aptitude and prohibited the use of group tests of aptitude in the schools. In 1975, Congress passed Public Law 94-142, the Education of All Handicapped Children Act. While the Act itself does not address testing, implementing regulations contained provisions for prohibiting the use of assessment instruments that were racially or culturally discriminatory. These and related efforts have had an effect on the practice of testing in the schools. Between 1975 and 1979, California imposed a statewide moratorium on using IQ tests in placing children in special education. School systems in a number of communities including New York City, Chicago, and Houston have curtailed or eliminated the use of standardized tests.

While such efforts have resulted in a more cautious, careful approach and, in some cases, have had a chilling effect on testing practices, their influence remains unclear. A review of the professional literature seems at first glance to support the notion of a decline in testing (Holt, 1967; Anastasi, 1967; Bersoff, 1973; Tolor, 1973; Cleveland, 1976). Many see this as a healthy, necessary retrenchment, needed to balance an enterprise that was oversold and abused by misuse (Bellack, 1971). Like all sciences in their youth, expectations were unrealistically high. Only as a science matures does it begin to better define its territory, clarifying its limits and capabilities.

Still, others question whether the decline has been more apparent than real. They point out that testing skills are still important prerequisites for the employment of psychologists (Levy and Fox, 1975). Some maintain that what actually may be occurring is a shift away from certain kinds of tests, while testing itself remains prominent (Ivnik, 1977). Finally, Sundberg et al. (1978) make this telling point: "even if the use of tests is declining, it cannot be concluded that assessment is declining."

The continuing need for assessment seems clear, since decision making is fundamental to many human endeavors. An effort to bring more scientific rigor and objectivity to the decision-making process seems inevitable. While the criticisms of tests are often social criticisms directed at how tests are used, the instruments themselves should be evaluated in terms of the principles of test construction, validity, and reliability. The fact remains that after decades of criticism, alternative methods proposed for decision making have not been shown to be more objective, valid, or reliable (Clarizio, 1979; Jensen, 1981).

WHAT IS NEEDED

This chapter has surveyed a wide range of issues, each of which has implications for the mental health and educational practices concerning children with emotional problems. Taken together, these issues provide a rationale for a systematic method of assessing, understanding, and helping children. What we have seen is the need for a system that:

1. Addresses the needs of a fairly large population of school-aged children who may be showing evidence of emotional adjustment difficulties, and specifically those with mild to moderate adjustment problems;
2. Addresses the needs of a growing number of children who are being forced to cope with rapid social change and disruptions in families and homes;
3. Is not bound by the restrictive categorical approach of traditional special education, but rather places emotional adjustment problems on a continuum of severity;
4. Provides a lower-level intervention to larger numbers of students than the psychological services typically available in the schools;

5. Incorporates a taxonomy of children's emotional disorders derived from empirical evidence and based on a theoretical model; and

6. Provides for both a descriptive and quantitative assessment of children that is valid, reliable, and clinically useful.

REFERENCES

Achenbach, T., and Edelbrock, C. The classification of child psychopathology: A review and analysis of empirical efforts. Psychol Bull, 1978, 85, 1275-1301.

Aiken, L. R. Psychological testing and assessment. Boston: Allyn & Bacon, 1976.

Allport, G. W., and Odbert, H. Trait names, a psycholexical study. Psychol Monogr, 1936, 47 (1).

Amrine, M. The 1965 congressional inquiry into testing: A commentary. Am Psychol, 1965, 20, 859-870.

Anastasi, A. Psychology, psychologists, and psychological testing. Am Psychol, 1967, 22, 297-305.

Ash, P. The implications of the Civil Rights Act of 1964 for psychological assessment in industry. Am Psychol, 1966, 21, 797-803.

Barack, R. Variables affecting the psychiatric hospitalization of children classified as emotionally disturbed. Unpublished doctoral dissertation, University of Pittsburgh, 1984.

Bellack, L. The TAT and CAT in clinical use. New York: Grune and Stratton, 1971.

Benton, M. The privacy invaders. New York: Cowen-McCann, 1964.

Bersoff, D. N. Silk purses into sow's ears: The decline of psychological testing and a suggestion for its redemption. Am Psychol, 1973, 28, 892-899.

Black, H. They shall not pass. New York: Random House, 1962.

Boyd, C. L. Training in individual testing at the University of Pittsburgh: 1904-1976. Unpublished manuscript, University of Pittsburgh, 1977.

Cattel, R. B. The description and measurement of personality. Yonkers-on-Hudson, N.Y.: World Book Co., 1946.

Clarizio, H. In defense of the IQ test. School Psychol Digest, 1979, 8, 79-88.

Clarizio, H. F., and McCoy, G. F. Behavior disorders of children. New York: Thomas Crowell Co., 1978.

Cleveland, S. Reflections on the rise of psychodiagnostics. Professional Psychology, 1976, 7, 309-318.

Cronbach, L. J. Essentials of psychological testing. 3rd ed. New York: Harper & Row, 1970.

Cronbach, L. J. Five decades of public controversy over mental testing. Am Psychol, 1975, 30, 1-14.

Downs, R. Molders of the modern mind. New York: Barnes and Noble, 1961.

Drake, E., and Shellenberger, S. Children of separation and divorce: A review of school programs and implications for the psychologist. School Psychol Rev, 1981, 10, 54-61.

Dreger, R. The children's behavioral classification project: An interim report. J Abnorm Child Psychol, 1977, 5, 289-297.

Edelbrock, C. Empirical classification of children's behavior disorders: Progress based on parent and teacher ratings. School Psychol Digest, 1979, 8, 355-369.

Eysenck, H. The dimensions of personality. London: Routledge and Paul, 1947.

Felner, R. S., Stolberg, A., and Cowen, E. L. Crisis events and school mental health referral patterns of young children. J Consult Clin Psychol, 1975, 43, 305-310.

Frank, L. K. Projective methods for the study of personality. J psychol, 1939, 8, 389-413.

Gilberstadt, H., and Duker, J. A handbook for clinical and actuarial MMPI interpretation. Philadelphia: W. B. Saunders, 1965.

Glick, P. C., and Norton, A. J. Marrying, divorcing and living together in the U.S. today. Population Bulletin, 1978, 32, 5. Washington, D.C.: Population Reference Bureau.

Graham, J. R. The MMPI: A practical guide. New York: Oxford University Press, 1977.

Gross, M. The brain watchers. New York: Random House, 1962.

Guidubaldi, J. Divorce research clarifies issues: A report on NASP's nationwide study. NASP Communiqué, 1983, 11, 1-7.

Guilford, J. P. Psychometric methods. New York: McGraw-Hill, 1954.

Hathaway, S. R. Personality inventories. In B. Wolman (Ed.), Handbook of clinical psychology. New York: McGraw-Hill, 1965.

Hetherington, E. M. Divorce: A child's perspective. Am Psychol, 1979, 34, 851-858.

Hoffman, B. The tyranny of testing. New York: Crowell-Collier, 1962.

Holt, R. Diagnostic testing: Present and future prospects. J Nerv Ment Dis, 1967, 144, 444-445.

Ivnick, R. J. The uncertain status of psychological tests in clinical psychology. Professional Psychology, 1977, 8, 206-213.

Jenkins, R. L. Psychiatric syndromes in children and their relation to family backgrounds. Am J Orthopsychiatry, 1966, 36, 450-457.

Jensen, A. Bias in mental testing. New York: The Free Press, 1981.

Johns, M. H., and Johns, B. Give your child a chance. Reston, Va.: Reston Pub. Co., 1982.

Kalter, N. Children of divorce in an outpatient psychiatric population. Am J Orthopsychiatry, 1977, 47, 40-51.

Kelly, J. B., and Wallerstein, J. S. Brief interventions with children in divorcing families. Am J Orthopsychiatry, 1977, 47, 23-36.

Lapouse, R., and Monk, M. An epidemiologic study of behavior characteristics in children. Am J Public Health, 1958, 48, 1134-1144.

Lapouse, R., and Monk, M. Fears and worries in a representative sample of children. Am J Orthopsychiatry, 1959, 29, 803-813.

Lanyon, R. E., and Goodstein, L. D. Personality assessment. 3rd ed. New York: Wiley, 1982.

Levy, M. R., and Fox, H. M. Psychological testing is alive and well. Professional Psychology, 1975, 6, 420-424.

Linden, K. W., and Linden, J. D. Modern mental measurement: A historical perspective. Boston: Houghton-Mifflin, 1968.

Lovell, V. R. The human use of personality tests: A dissenting view. Am Psychol, 1967, 22, 383-393.

Marks, P. A., and Seeman, W. Actuarial description of abnormal personality. Baltimore: Williams and Wilkins, 1983.

McDermott, J. F. Divorce and its psychiatric sequelae in children. Arch Gen Psychiatry, 1970, 23, 421-427.

Meehl, P. E. Clinical versus statistical prediction: A theoretical analysis and review of the evidence. University of Minnesota Press, 1954.

Meehl, P. E. Wanted--a good cookbook. Am Psychol, 1956, 11, 263-272.

Mezzich, J. E. Patterns and issues in multiaxial psychiatric diagnosis. Psychol Med, 1979, 9, 125-137.

Morgan, C. D., and Murray, H. A. A method for investigating fantasies: The Thematic Apperception Test. Arch Neurol Psychiatry, 1935, 34, 289-306.

New York State Department of Mental Hygiene. Mental health research unit report. Albany, N.Y.: New York State, 1974.

Packard, V. The hidden persuaders. New York: McKay, 1957.

Quay, H. C. A dimensional approach to behavior disorder: The Revised Behavior Problem Checklist. School Psychol Rev, 1983, 12, 244-249.

Reynolds, M. C., and Birch, J. W. Teaching exceptional children in all America's schools. Reston, Va.: Council on Exceptional Children, 1977.

Sattler, J. M. Assessment of children's intelligence and special abilities. 2nd ed. Boston: Allyn and Bacon, 1982.

Spitzer, R. L., Williams, J. B., and Skodol, A. E. DSM-III: The major achievements and an overview. Am J Psychiatry, 1980, 137, 151-163.

Sundberg, N. D., Snowden, L. R., and Reynolds, W. M. Toward assessment of personal competence and incompetence in life situations. Ann Rev Psychol, 1978, 29, 179-221.

Thurstone, L. L. Primary mental abilities. Chicago: University of Chicago Press, 1938.

Tolor, A. Diagnosing the state of the diagnostic function: An analysis of the literature. J Clin Psychol, 1973, 29, 338-342.

Werry, J. S., and Quay, H. C. The prevalence of behavior symptoms in younger elementary school children. Am J Orthopsychiatry, 1971, 41, 136-143.

Weston, A. F. Privacy and freedom. New York: Atheneum, 1967.

2

SOURCES OF STRESS

THE STUDY OF STRESS

Stress is a term that comes to the social sciences through biology from engineering, where it applies to physical forces exerted on objects or structures. It began to be used in the biological sciences to describe the phenomena of strong emotions affecting physiological functioning, as had been reported by physiologists such as W. B. Cannon (1871-1945).

During early fluoroscopic studies of the digestive mechanisms of animals, Cannon had observed that the stomach movements of his subjects ceased when they were emotionally excited. These observations led him to examine the effects of strong emotions on bodily functioning in a series of studies conducted between 1911 and 1915. Subsequently, he was able to observe the effects of physical and psychological trauma when, as a member of a committee formed to study trauma shock, he visited the casualty clearing stations on the battlefields of France, during World War I. Probably Cannon's best known contribution was his coining of the term "homeostatis" which he used to describe the mechanism of autonomous adjustment within the organism that sought to restore equilibrium after a disruption. He popularized that concept in his classic work Wisdom of the Body, published in 1932.

Cannon's experiences reflected the two main concerns of early studies of stress: (1) the effect of the emotions on physiological functioning, and (2) the impact of specific traumatic events, such as wars, disasters, and so on. While work continued in the psychophysiological aspects, the focus increasingly shifted to the study of traumatic events. That shift was impelled by the experience of two world wars.

In Europe, Sigmund Freud, observing the returning veterans of World War I, became interested in the psychic trauma of combat. He pointed to the many similarities between the victims of "shell shock," and those of accidents and disasters (Freud, 1928). Followers of Freud and others were later to study the psychological stress associated with war (Grinker and Spiegel, 1945; Kardiner and Spiegel, 1947), family disruption (Freud and Burlingham, 1943), accidents and disasters (Janis, 1962; Kinston and Rosser, 1974), and concentration camp experiences (Bettelheim, 1960).

From a psychoanalytic viewpoint, the unpleasant emotional experience associated with such danger situations could be seen as a type of anxiety. By 1926, Freud had distinguished between two types of anxiety. In threatening situations, signal anxiety arose as a warning. As such, it always implied an outer referent. But there was also a more basic, internal, instinctual anxiety. This was the type commonly associated with neuroses. Recognizing this distinction in a review of psychoanalytic theories of anxiety, Compton (1980) proposes that further study be given to the question, "What is the relationship between sensory perceptions associated with painful stimuli, and the sensations of internal disequilibrium or 'need'?"

The notion that anxiety might be of two types, as proposed by Freud and reiterated by Compton, finds similar expression in the work of Henry Murray. Murray based his formulations about personality on psychoanalytic principles (1938). He stressed that a personality theory must consider the organism and its milieu taken together. He emphasized the dynamics of the person-environment unit, and characterized the kind of effect the stimulus situation had upon the organism as an environmental tendency or press. The press could bring the threat of harm or the possibility of benefit to the organism. Murray further maintained that behavioral trends might be motivated by a drive or need within the individual. Thus the individual might be motivated by need, press, or some need-press combination. While Murray's views were strongly influenced by psychoanalytic theory, it was in the area of motivational psychology that he made a most unique contribution, and his influence on the development of personality assessment methods has been considerable (Ruitenbeek, 1964).

Throughout the 1920s and 1930s research into stress proceeded along the two established lines, physiological and trauma studies. It was only after World War II that stress began gradually to be seen in a wider psychosocial context. One impetus for this wider application came from the work of another physiologist, Hans Selye.

In his book The Stress of Life (1956), Selye reported on tissue studies of endocrine glands. In these studies, he observed and measured tissue changes such as adrenal enlargement and lymphatic atrophy, which he saw as stress manifestations. Relating his work to the findings of physiological research linking specific changes with stress, Selye sought a unifying stress theory. He proposed a definition of stress as a state manifested by a syndrome consisting of nonspecific induced changes within a biologic system. He saw the organism's generalized response, which he called the general adaptation syndrome, as a stress syndrome. For Selye adaptation was a key concept. Life, he maintained, was largely a process of adaptation. It was through the general adaptation syndrome that various internal organs helped man to adapt to the constant changes in his environment. Although Selye's theory was grounded in biology, it was the psychosomatic and psychological implications of his work that were to stimulate considerable interest in the subject of stress.

Throughout the 1950s and 1960s stress began to be increasingly studied in a broader psychosocial context. No longer limited to the rather narrow association with traumatic events, an awareness was growing that stress was ubiquitous. It was, as Selye had reminded us, an inevitable part of life. Gradually, a psychosocial perspective on stress was being developed as various interactionist models were proposed (Endler, 1982).

From this perspective, stress is seen as arising from the interaction between the person and his situation. Endler and Magnusson (1976) have presented four basic postulates of interactional psychology: (1) behavior is a function of a continuous and bidirectional process of person-situation interaction; (2) the individual is an intentional, active agent in this process; (3) motivational, emotional, and cognitive variables play important determining roles on the person's side; and (4) the psychological meaning that the situation has for the person is an essential determining factor of behavior.

Other workers were to emphasize the cognitive variables that gave psychological meaning to events and situations that might help to determine the stress associated with them (Arnold, 1960). Lazarus (1976) conceptualized stress as a problem arising out of a demand that taxes the system composed of the individual and his environment. A key role is played by the cognitive appraisal of the demand by the individual. Primary cognitive appraisal is the mental process of evaluating an event in terms of its significance for one's well-being (Lazarus and Launier, 1978). A judgment is made whether the event constitutes a threat with the possibility of harm or loss as a consequence (Coyne and Lazarus, 1980).

These issues led researchers to investigate the stimulus properties that might make it stressful, and the appraisal process which could be seen as a means of mediating the stressfulness of the stimulus. Other properties of the individual and the situation that might serve as mediators of stress also were being identified and examined. There was an interest in the response to stress, the coping skills employed in adapting. Finally, there was continued interest in the effects of stress, emotional, behavioral, and physical.

Even as the study of stress evolved from a concern with specific traumatic events to more general psychosocial situations, physiological and psychosomatic research was also expanding. The role of stress in the etiology of various illnesses and diseases became the subject of intensive study. The role of stress in cancer (Achtenberg, Simonton, and Simonton, 1976), ulcers (Cobb and Rose, 1973), heart disease and hypertension (Wheatley, 1981), and a number of other physical problems, was examined. As the debilitating effects of excessive stress became better understood, interest grew in techniques developed to manage and reduce stress.

This most recent interest arose from the findings of research conducted in the 1960s that involuntary autonomic functions could be altered by certain conditioning techniques (Miller, 1969). One such technique employed biofeedback to help the individual gain control over aspects of autonomic functioning by providing him with ongoing information about functions like heartbeat, galvanic skin response level, and muscular tension. By monitoring these functions and making conscious attempts to alter them, changes could be effected.

Along with biofeedback techniques, there was a renewed interest in progressive relaxation, a technique originally advocated by Jacobson in the 1930s. Jacobson (1938), noting that emotional problems were often associated with skeletal tension, reasoned that muscular relaxation might have a positive effect. He suggested that with conscious attention and practice an individual could learn progressive relaxation. More recently, it was found that biofeedback could be used to induce muscular relaxation, and thus reduce various symptoms associated with psychological stress. Stoyva and Andersen (1982), in a recent review of the subject, concluded that "a major practical consequence of developments in biofeedback has been the demonstration of the clinical usefulness of relaxation training, a fact of central significance for stress management" (p. 752).

A review of the history of stress research leaves one with two general impressions of the concept of stress: (1) it has a certain intuitive appeal, and (2) it is vague and overly inclusive (Apply and Trumbull, 1967). Yet it may be the very elasticity of the concept that gives it much of its intuitive appeal and utility in psychosocial applications. Lerner (1982) recognized that when he said, "a lot of the fuzziness about the concept of stress is what makes it so valuable." He goes on to quote Aristotle to the effect that it is always an error to try to make a science more exacting than its subject allows for. This warning seems particularly important for workers in the social sciences. Nevertheless, some definition is called for if subsequent activities like identification, observation, assessment, and measurement are to be conducted in the scientific study of stress.

From the perspective taken in this book, psychological stress may be defined as a state of emotional tension arising from two main conditions: failure of the environment to meet the needs of the individual, or events or situations which the individual perceives as threatening. Seen in this way stress is a stimulus (McGrath, 1970). It can act as a drive or motivator (Farber, 1955), as the individual, seeking drive reduction, responds in adaptive or maladaptive ways.

STRESSFUL LIFE EVENTS AND SITUATIONS

One class of stressors which has received considerable research attention are the ordinary and extraordinary changes that an individual may encounter in life. Initially, the focus was on extraordinary events, those which might disrupt ongoing activities and bring significant change. The trauma studies might be considered in that category. Events such as natural and man-made disasters were the original stressful life events (SLEs). With the broadening perspective on stress, studies of potentially stressful life events began to include events of a lesser magnitude of impact, such as divorce, moves and relocations, job loss. These were the more ordinary events which most individuals might expect to experience in the course of a lifetime.

As has been pointed out, the experience of two world wars in the first half of the twentieth century focused attention on the effects of massive trauma. While occasional single case studies had been reported in the early literature (compare James' [1911] personal account of his reactions to the San Francisco earthquake), systematic studies of disaster began to appear with some frequency following World War II.

Kinston and Rosser (1974) reviewed the studies of the effects of disaster, which they defined as situations of collective massive stress. After examining studies on war, concentration camp experiences, earthquakes, tornados, fires, and explosions, they detailed the many psychological reactions to stress including denial of the threat; terror and elation; invulnerability and helplessness; dazed, stunned, and bewildered behavior; and childlike regression.

There are fewer studies of children in disaster; however, some conclusions have been forthcoming. Some of the earliest studies involving children were carried out in England during World War II when many children were separated from their parents by wartime evacuation precautions. Anna Freud and her colleagues reported that while acute disturbance was common, it was often transient; however, the separation could have longer lasting effects. In addition, they found that children reacted more strongly to maternal emotions than to the explosions of bombs, suggesting the key role that could be played by the parents.

Silber, Perry, and Bloch (1957) have also emphasized the important role played by the parent as a mediator of the stressful event. In their study of children who experienced a tornado, they concluded that some parents were better able to assist their children to cope by helping them to integrate the experience. Fostering verbalization, for example, was one technique which they felt helped children to avoid more serious emotional disturbance. Also more effective were those parents who provided support during and after the disaster, who allowed some regression, and who held realistic expectations of the child's ability to recover.

Blaufarb and Levine (1972) reported on a crisis intervention program for parents and children set up in the aftermath of an earthquake in California in 1971. They worked with parents to reestablish the family as a unit, and help them to reassert themselves as the guiding and steadying influence in the family. The intervention directed toward children involved encouraging them to verbalize about their fears, thoughts, and feelings after the experience.

Newman (1976) studied children who were the survivors of the Buffalo Creek flood. She suggested that the effects on children could be attributed to three major factors: (1) the developmental level of children at the time of the disaster, (2) their perspective of the family's reaction, and (3) their direct exposure to the disaster. She concluded that children form their own theory of a disaster based on their own reactions and their perceptions of the reactions of their parents and other adults.

Kinston and Rosser (1974), in discussing children's reactions, make an interesting distinction by dividing them into initial reactions and later posttraumatic responses seen in the aftermath of the disaster. They summarize the initial reaction to disaster this way:

> In the early phases of disaster their reactions are a function of the way in which reality filters down to them and so they mirror their parents' reactions rather than relating directly to the event. The most predominant fear at all ages is separation from the parents. If this does not occur, and if the parents cope with the situation, children may show little awareness of danger and minimal anxiety (p. 445).

The later posttraumatic responses included: a compulsive working over of the disaster and associated scenes in play or dreams along with fears of recurrence. The general conclusion was that, in the aftermath of disaster, children rarely needed specialized help, but they could benefit from the opportunity to discuss their fears with a sympathetic adult.

The study of the more ordinary life events has been traced to Adolf Meyer's (1866–1950) work at the turn of the century (Dohrenwend and Dohrenwend, 1974). Meyer was a Swiss physician who, after immigrating to America in 1890, worked in a number of state hospitals. Through his work he became convinced of the importance of collecting life history data on patients. Later, as head of the New York State Pathological Institute, he established standards and procedures for the systematic collection of data, including information on the patient's home, family, and life situation. He suggested the use of a "life chart" to facilitate data collection. Such a device would list "changes of habitat, of school entrance, graduations or changes or failures; the various jobs; the dates of important births and deaths in the family, and other fundamental important environmental influences" (Lief, 1948, p. 420).

Modern interest in SLEs is due largely to the important contributions of Thomas Holmes and his associates begun in the 1950s (Holmes and Rahe, 1967; Holmes and Masuda, 1974; Holmes, 1979). They adopted Meyer's idea of the life chart as a means of systematically collecting data on patients that would allow a detailed examination of their lives in prospective and retrospective investigations of illness. They attempted to develop a life chart device to study the quality and quantity of those events which were empirically observed to cluster near the time of the illness. This list was composed of events that have significance in American society, such as marriage, trouble with the boss, death of a spouse, and so on. They included in their list not only those that might normally be seen as negatively stressful, but also those that might be socially desirable, following a definition of stress as arising from events which disrupt equilibrium (Garmezy, 1981) and require some adjustment on the part of the individual.

Holmes and his colleagues constructed their list after reviewing more than 5,000 case histories for significant events. The resulting Schedule of Recent Experience (SRE) was used to gather data on the frequency of occurrence of various life events. Later, they were to propose a psychophysical method of scaling life events by assigning them weighted values based on the individual's perception of how much life change was associated with each event.

In an effort to estimate the magnitude of the events, 394 subjects were presented with a questionnaire based on the SRE. An arbitrary value of 500 was assigned to marriage as a benchmark. Subjects were then asked to rate each event relative to the amount of adjustment necessary to marriage. For convenience, the resulting mean values for each item were divided by ten, and called "Life Change Units." These data allowed them to construct an instrument, the Social Readjustment Rating Scale (SRRS), which contained 43 life events observed to occur prior to the onset of illness, along with estimates of the magnitude of each event, expressed in Life Change Units.

The SRRS has become one of the most widely used instruments in the study of SLEs. Studies have been reported linking mounting life change and sudden cardiac death (Rahe and Lind, 1971), and time of onset of myocardial infarction (Rahe and Paasikivi, 1971). Holmes and Masuda (1974) have reported a direct relationship between the magnitude of life crisis and the risk of health change.

In addition to studies of the relationship between SLEs and diseases and illness, Holmes and Masuda (1974) have reported on a series of studies that explored cross-cultural implications by examining the relative magnitude assigned to the events by subjects in various countries.

The work of Holmes and his associates has stimulated considerable interest in SLEs, and a number of basic questions have been raised:

<u>How can SLEs be defined and identified?</u>

While most writers might agree that stressful life events are those that necessitate some adjustment on the part of the individual, some have focused on those that are generally seen as negative experiences (thus equating stress with distress), while others have taken the broader view that would include even those usually seen as positive. In addition, in order to identify potentially stressful events, some knowledge of the population being studied is necessary. While some events occur with greater frequency in a given culture, investigators have found that the frequencies of others vary widely among specific groups within a population. As a result, some have proposed that various life events inventories be developed with events relevant to particular populations (Hurst, 1979).

How can the magnitude of SLEs be estimated?

The problelm of scaling a life events list raises a number of methodological issues. As we have seen, Holmes chose to estimate the amount of readjustment necessary as rated by subjects who were asked to draw on their personal experience. Other researchers have asked subjects to rate the amount of stress, distress, or upset associated with various events (Paykel, Prusoff, and Uhlenhuth, 1971; Paykel and Uhlenhuth, 1972; Horowitz, Schaefer, and Cooney, 1974; Chandler, 1981). While Hurst (1979) has found high correlations between these two methods, he cautions that what is rated might make a difference in the comparisons an investigator makes and the conclusions he draws. The related issue of who is the preferred rater, for example, one who has experienced or is experiencing an event, or a more objective observer, continues to be debated.

What is the relationship among SLEs, that is, how can they be conceptualized, classified, or clustered?

Many ways of clustering SLEs have been proposed based on a priori relationships. For example, Paykel et al. (1971) classified events as exit or entrance events. Kaplan (1980) maintains that life events reflect either continuity or changes which are not easily predicted. He therefore proposes classifying events as normative or nonnormative. Dohrenwend (1979) classified events as extreme (to illustrate, man-made or natural disasters) or more ordinary (for example, divorce). He then further sorted the latter into three subtypes: (1) loss of loved one, (2) severe illness and injury, and (3) events that disrupt social supports. Dohrenwend has also proposed that events might be classified accerding to locus of control, that is, those over which the individual has some control versus those over which he has no control. In this context, events under the individual's control might be seen as ineffective attempts to cope (and thus secondary stressors) with some more primary stressor--one that is outside of his control.

Each proposed scheme seems open to problems of interpretation since disagreements could arise regarding which events might be included in one group or another.

However, classification schemes based on a priori theoretical assumptions are not the only type available. Statistical techniques may be used to examine the relationships that exist within a body of data. Hurst (1979), in discussing the classification issue, advocates the use of cluster analysis to identify groups of events with common effects on individuals. Hoesch (1983) used a factor analytic technique to examine the data derived from a children's life events inventory. She found four significant factors, which she labeled as (1) marital issues, (2) school-related problems, (3) family arguments, and (4) family troubles.

What is the relationship between SLEs and various psychological and physical problems?

This question addresses the primary rationale for the SLE studies. Many studies have examined that relationship to try to ascertain what contribution SLEs might have toward later mental disorder (Barrett, 1979). While some correlation has been found between SLEs and certain psychological problems, the question of causality remains unanswered. Do SLEs cause extreme reactions? Are the reactions themselves sources of stress? Are SLEs and psychological problems both caused by some third factor or group of factors? For example, in the case of divorce, is it that divorce causes stress or are there more fundamental causes, perhaps personality factors, which may precipitate divorce and impair the individual's ability to cope with that event?

While ordinary life events might be expected to affect children's functioning, the subject was probably first investigated because of the belief that childhood experiences have a considerable impact on later development. Brown's (1979) findings that the loss of a mother before age 11 acts as a vulnerability factor to increase the risk of depression is typical of that reasoning. Langer and Michael (1963) maintain that no single stress or combination of stresses is so great a statistical risk to adult mental health as is an accumulation of stressful factors in childhood, the risk being directly proportional to the number of such factors. In order to investigate this problem, longitudinal studies are necessary.

Such a longitudinal study was described by Moore and his colleagues (Moore, Hindley, and Falkner, 1954; Moore, 1959) at the Centre for Human Development in

England. These researchers followed a group of subjects from before birth to adolescence, investigating the consequences of such potentially stressful experiences as temporary separations of various kinds, the birth of a sibling, change of home, divided daily care, and others. In addition, they examined certain conditions at and before birth, which might help to determine the individual's reactions to such experiences. Such longitudinal studies will provide a better understanding of those factors that might contribute to increased susceptibility to stress.

Another approach, analogous to that taken by researchers with adults, was to study the role of SLEs in predicting children's physical problems. Mutter and Schleifer (1966) examined the histories of hospitalized children by conducting a semi-structured interview with their parents, in order to obtain information on life events and family interactions that occurred within the six-month period preceding the onset of somatic illness. When matched with a healthy control group, the hospitalized group showed a significantly greater number of changes in their psychosocial setting. In addition, significantly more children with somatic illness had experienced actual and/or threatened loss than had the healthy children. Differences in socioeconomic status and neighborhood social structure were not found to be significant factors.

Further support for the role of life events as etiological factors in the diseases of children came from Coddington and his colleagues (Coddington, 1972; Heisel, Raitz, Ream, Rappaport, and Coddington, 1973). They also found that discriminations could be made between hospitalized children and their healthy peers based on the number of SLEs that they had experienced. Data on life events that had occurred prior to the onset of illness with children with rheumatoid arthritis, general pediatric patients, surgical patients, and psychiatric patients were compared with data on normal healthy children. They found that children with illnesses had experienced significantly more frequent and/or severe life events than did healthy children.

In the course of their investigations these researchers developed several lists of SLEs for use with children and adolescents. Coddington (1972) modified the SRE to include items relevant to the lives of children. He developed separate lists for preschool, elementary, junior high, and senior high school students. Following the procedures used by Holmes, he chose one item, "birth of brother or sister," to be arbitrarily assigned a value of 500. He then asked a group of teachers and mental health professionals to rate the items relevant to the benchmark event.

Again, following Holmes' procedures, Coddington calculated life change units (LCUs) for each event. Various groups of raters with differing professional identities and experience in direct work with children were generally found to agree in their opinions regarding the relative amount of readjustment associated with the various events.

The resulting lists, compiled for the various school age groups, could be used by parents who were asked to indicate those experiences that had occurred to their child during the preceding year. Coddington found that LCU scores increased with age, while there was no significant effect due to race or social class on the scores.

Coddington's list served as the basis for further studies concerned with SLEs of children, and in the process several modifications of his list were proposed.

Sandler and his colleagues (Sandler and Block, 1979; Sandler, 1980; Sandler and Ramsey, 1980) modified Coddington's list for elementary school children in an effort to examine the relationship between stress and the adaptation of children in kindergarten through third grade. The resulting measure was a 32-item schedule which included 25 items adopted from Coddington's list, five items taken from a schedule of recent events used in a previous study (Gersten, Langner, Eisenberg, and Simcha-Fagan, 1977), and two items added by the authors. All items were rated as either desirable or undesirable, and all items selected were those deemed to be outside of the child's control. The latter restriction was imposed so that items that might be seen as a consequence of the child's behavioral adjustment would be eliminated from the list.

Items could be scored by their social desirability or by the weighted scores derived by Coddington. Parents were asked to indicate those events that had occurred to their child during the previous year. When compared with data on the children's classroom adjustment and behavior, the authors were able to demonstrate a relationship between recent SLEs and the adjustment of young elementary school children (Sandler and Block, 1979).

Chandler (1981) has proposed another modification of Coddington's list. In developing a list of events for clinical use, he proposed eliminating from Coddington's list for elementary school-age children those items that might have desirable connotations (for example, personal achievement), as well as those of relatively low incidence (for example, discovery of being an adopted child). He also proposed adding some school-related items (for example, learning problems, need for special education). In all, ten items from Coddington's original 36 were deleted and 11 were added. The resulting Children's Life Events Inventory contained 37 events of elementary school-age children, usually associated with some degree of negative stress, that could be completed by parents during clinical interviews. Because of the long-term effects of some events, parents are asked to indicate all the events that have occurred from birth until the present.

A procedure suggested by Paykel (1973) was selected as an alternative method for scaling the events. To demonstrate the method, Paykel and his associates provided subjects with a list of life events, and asked each to indicate how upsetting the event would be. A simple 0 to 20 rating scale, assuming equal intervals, was used. This loose scaling concept was chosen because of its connotations of upset and discomfort. The findings were similar to those obtained by Holmes and Rahe (1967), and the scaling technique proved to be feasible, with a remarkably high agreement across different sociodemographic groups. The authors then ranked the events by mean scores in descending order of magnitude (Paykel, Prusoff, and Uhlenhuth, 1971).

The use of weighted scores, derived from consensual judgment, has caused some debate, especially regarding whether such weighted scores offer an advantage over a simple frequency count of the number of events. Rahe and Arthur (1978), noting the high correlations between weighted and unweighted totals, see little value in going beyond the mere counting of reported events. On the other hand, it has been argued that when events are aggregated over an entire list in the same way for all individuals, both weighted and unweighted scores should be tested, and the former, simpler scores adopted if the two approaches yield similar results (Dohrenwend, Kransoff, Askenasy, and Dohrenwend, 1982; Lorimor, Justice, McBee, and Weinman, 1979). Mulvey (1979) lends support to this approach in a study of age differences with recent life events experience. He found that the number of events experienced in one year did not vary with age, nor did the weighted scores differ. The average weight of events reported by individuals, however, was found to vary, increasing significantly with age.

Following Paykel's procedure, Chandler (1981) requested that a group of teachers and mental health professionals rate the events according to the average degree of stress associated with each. The resulting mean scores were used to rank the events. As in the previous studies, considerable agreement was found between the groups as to the relative severity of the stress associated with each event.

As some consensus developed on the SLEs of children, studies began to examine their effects on children's mental health (Gersten, Langner, Eisenberg, and Orzeck, 1974), and on school performance and classroom behavior (Boike, Gesten, Cowen, Felner, and Francis, 1978; Felner, Ginter, Boike, and Cowen, 1981; Gesten, Scher, and Cowen, 1978; Rolf and Garmezy, 1974; Sandler, 1980; Sandler and Block, 1979; Siegel, 1981). For example, Felner, Stollberg, and Cowen (1975) found that 20 percent of the children identified by teachers as having adjustment problems had a history that included either divorce/separation or death of a parent.

SLEs have been found to discriminate between groups of children with adjustment problems and normal, control groups (Sandler and Ramsey, 1980; Felner et al., 1975; Sandler and Block, 1979). More recently, investigators have included the history of SLEs as one element in defining populations of high-risk children (Egeland, Schakel, Erikson, Rahe, and Mathieu, 1982).

While the study of life events as stressors necessitates some identification of, and agreement on, those events which may be potentially stressful, the perception which the individual holds of various events remains crucial in determining whether a given event will be stressful for that individual. Haan (1982) spoke to this point when she stated that no listing of objective stress stimuli was likely to be satisfactory because "stress is the result of a situation having a certain meaning" (p. 256).

Researchers have consistently emphasized the key role of perception. Endler (1975), for example, sees the perception of situational interpersonal threat as determining the extent of anxiety in a given situation. Lazarus (1981) has also emphasized the central role of cognitive appraisal in threat, loss, or harm situations.

Magnusson (1982), in discussing the situational aspects of stress, distinguishes between the actual environment and the perceived environment. He sees early stress research, strongly influenced by behaviorism, as concerned with the actual environment. He goes on to point out that the research on life events and their stressful effects has been strongly affected by theories dealing with the moderating effects of perceived social supports, perceived prediction and control, and so on (Sarason and Sarason, 1981). As Magnusson (1982) explains,

> This [perceived environment] approach has been particularly important in interactional personality theory. And this view has greatly influenced research in stress and anxiety. It has changed the focus from an interest in how external stimulation per se provokes emotional, physiological, and behavioral anxiety reactions to an interest in how stress reactions are elicited by expectations about the consequences of stressful conditions (p. 232).

Following Magnusson's suggestion, it would be appropriate in identifying stressors that arise from the environment, to examine both the actual and the perceived environments.

The last source of stress to be discussed is unfulfilled inner needs. While it has long been recognized that individuals respond to stimuli in the environment, there also has been considerable attention given, in motivational theory, to actions resulting from unmet, or only partially satisfied, needs (Freud, 1928; Lewin, 1935; Maslow, 1954; Murphy, 1956; Murray, 1938). These theorists, particularly those who espouse a dynamic view of human motivation, maintain, as Murray (1938) put it, "that the organism and its milieu must be considered together" in a dynamic interaction. Murray, reacting to the contemporary interest in drive theory (compare Tolman, 1932), warned of limiting the study of motivation to the external determinants of behavior. Rather, he proposed that theorists study each episode, a single creature-environment interaction, as the endurance of a certain kind of press in conjunction with a certain kind of need. Behavioral trends could be attributed to a hypothetical force within the organism (a need), to an environmental press, or to some combination of the two.

The interactive aspect of need was summarized by Maddi (1968):

> Take as an example the need for affiliation. The inner state may be specific cognitive and affective conditions best described as loneliness. This loneliness may be initiating in the sense that it exists regardless of whether the actual environmental circumstances are so affiliatively depriving. Or it may be reacting, in the sense that it must be aroused by affiliatively depriving circumstances. Regardless of whether the circumstances are or are not depriving, they must be perceived by the person as being so (p. 246).

Maddi goes on to point out that when aroused, needs exist as tension states that lead to instrumental behavior.

One of Murray's major contributions was his taxonomy of needs, some of which related to survival, while others were more psychosocial in nature. Murray's list included many of the needs that would be widely utilized and researched by subsequent workers including dominance, autonomy, aggression, sex, achievement, affiliation, and nurturance.

SPECIAL CONSIDERATIONS OF CHILDHOOD

In addition to the specific instances of stress associated with potentially stressful life events, there are two other major sources of childhood stress: normal developmental stresses, and endemic general social stress. Table 2.1 outlines the major sources of childhood stress.

Normal Developmental Stresses

Child development workers have long recognized two levels or modes of thinking, sometimes called magical and realistic. Kessler (1966) points out that this is similar to Freud's distinction between the pleasure principle (primary process thinking) and the reality principle (secondary process thinking). Freud illustrated primary process thinking by the dream in which anything was possible, often in defiance of logic. Gradually the more realistic secondary processes begin to dominate the child's mental activity, although lapses or regressions to more primitive primary process thinking continue throughout life. The difference between the magical and realistic perceptions of the world is a major cause of misunderstanding between the adult's and the child's perception of the same event.

TABLE 2.1

Major Sources and Examples of Childhood Stress

Normal Developmental Stresses

--From meeting reality demands
--From differences in adult and child perceptions

Endemic (general, social/environmental) Stress

--Social trends affecting attitudes of parents toward children
--Social trends affecting sexual roles and sexual identity

Specific (crises) Stressors

--Divorce
--Hospitalization
--Learning problems

Examples of magical thinking abound in the developmental literature on young children. It has been observed that young children adopt the notion that they can magically influence events by an application of will. This notion can result in considerable guilt if they wish someone harm and a mishap occurs. Similarly, young children are likely to feel that their thoughts are readily apparent to adults, and this might result in considerable confusion and uncertainty in the child. Placing magical thinking in the context of the adult real world sets the stage for inevitable misunderstanding, frustration, and conflict.

The inconsistencies in perception can be important in the etiology of emotional disorders. Kessler (1966) relates these inconsistencies to symptom formation:

> A symptom originates from affective needs rather than logic and it usually contains within it a kernel of irrational thinking . . . some object . . . has become invested with all kinds of extra meanings beyond the realistic or logical.

The dissonance in perception may be seen when the child, in appraising some event or situation, perceives the threat of harm or loss. If this perception results from primitive thinking, it may well be that an observing adult would characterize the child's perception as unrealistic. Nevertheless, the child adopts a stress response in an effort to cope with the perceived stress. A clinical vignette might serve to illustrate this sort of problem.

David

David is a six-year-old first grader who was brought to the clinic by his mother. He had a history of bedwetting and generally immature behavior. Recently, he had been having problems in school coping with his work. His teachers had described him as a child who tries hard but has trouble completing his work. A family history showed that David's sister had been badly burned in a fire when he was two and a half years old. Subsequently his parents had to spend an inordinate amount of time with his sister taking her for frequent treatment at the burn clinic, with the inevitable result that they had less time to spend with David. Apparently David interpreted this sudden loss of parental attention as rejection, and the threat of further rejection caused him considerable stress. In an effort to cope, David had adopted a regressive, immature, and dependent response style.

This example illustrates the differences between adult reality and the child's interpretation of that reality. While the adults saw the necessity of intensive treatment of the child, the sibling saw only rejection.

Jean Piaget (1951) was to spend a lifetime studying the differences in thinking between adults and children. In explaining how children struggle with causal relationships, he introduced the concept of phenomenalistic causality, that is, the belief that when two events occur in succession the first "causes" the second (Elkind, 1976). The child's use of phenomenalistic causality lays the groundwork for confusion, misunderstanding, and miscommunication between adult and child, and thus becomes a potential source of stress. In a similar way, other properties of the immature mental processes of children such as conceptual understanding, developing controls and egocentrism, all represent potential sources of stress.

Piaget (1951) carefully studied the conceptual differences between children and adults. He found that concepts of space and time consistent with adult reality were lacking in children. As a result a child's view, for example, of a tolerable delay in waiting for some reward or treat may differ markedly from the adult's, resulting in a situation that generates considerable stress.

In a similar way the amount of impulse control available to children is limited by their level of maturity. Since they have less control over their behavior than adults, they are more likely to behave impulsively, to act out, and to press the limits of a social situation that might require restraint and control. Once again, this characteristic of immaturity may bring them into conflict with adults.

Egocentrism is yet another characteristic mode that dominates the thinking of young children. Egocentrism colors their world view, as they perceive objects and other individuals in terms of the self-referent. Since young children are unable to take another's point of view, they fail to perceive social demands. The child, trying to gain his mother's attention, may be unaware of her needs, competing demands on her time, or her desire for activities where he might be legitimately excluded. As a result his behavior may seem insensitive or perverse, and parental discipline may be forthcoming. Frequent troubles between children and adults stem from these differences in world view.

The final source of stress is found in the normal course of human development. Development involves change, and change is often stressful. Sometimes the changes in the developing child are sudden and dramatic; at other times they are more gradual and subtle.

Erikson (1964, 1968) in his theory of development, sees the process as a series of potential crises. A crisis is a time of increased vulnerability to a particular psychosocial problem. Successful resolution of these crises fosters development and contributes to the healthy, growing personality. Erikson describes five developmental crises during childhood and adolescence.

The first crisis occurs in infancy, and is labeled as "trust versus mistrust." It may be that the infant's first experience of stress occurs when physical needs are not immediately met. Crying does not bring an immediate response from mother. The tension that arises as a result of that delay serves as a prototype for later stress arising from unmet needs. A basic trust of the environment (and significant others) can develop if needs are reasonably met. Feeding, touching, loving, caring, and attending to the child's needs foster the sense of trust.

The second crisis is what Erikson has called "autonomy versus shame and doubt." This occurs in early childhood, as the child begins to test his control over his environment. At this stage the toddler has the first opportunity to exert some independence. As he ventures forth to explore, there is the inevitable separation from the mother. If stress is associated with this initial attempt at separation, it is likely that later life events that involve separation, like going to school, leaving home, and marriage, will also be highly stressful for the individual. If the child is not allowed to achieve some degree of separation, a sense of shame and doubt in one's capabilities could result. On the other hand, if the child is able to achieve some initial emancipation from the mother, a sense of autonomy may be gained.

The crisis of "initiative versus guilt" occurs at around four to five years of age. Initiative results from a developing sense of purpose, curiosity, and ambition. The parents may deny the child permission to explore certain places or to engage in some activities. Their prohibitions are important in forming the child's conscience. Unusually restrictive adults may block initiative, frustrate and inhibit the child, and engender a sense of guilt.

The crisis of "accomplishment versus inferiority" provides a theme for much of the child's school years (ages six through 11 years). Intellectual curiosity and performance dominate the child who learns by doing. Since the sense of accomplishment is so intimately bound with the emerging self-image, disruptions in learning can have damaging effects by engendering feelings of inadequacy and inferiority. Accordingly, learning difficulties in school are a major source of stress at this age.

Learning requires certain preconditions and a readiness on the part of the learner. For a child, readiness involves a degree of development in physical, psychoneuro-

In times of inner doubt and uncertainty one may turn to others for confirmation. Because self-doubt and uncertainty are so chronic in adolescence, the need for others to approve is particularly strong. The group of adolescents thus becomes a mutually reinforcing circle, defined by social mannerisms that support group identity. There is a strong devotion to the tastes, interests, clothes, music, and language of the group. Popularity and acceptance become important goals, and exclusion and rejection the painful consequences of failure.

Group membership always requires some sacrifice of individuality. Assuring a place in the group may mean violating some norm, personal, parental, or legal. This creates another set of problems, since it requires submerging one's individual identity in the interests of group membership. Since the adolescent depends on group membership to assist in his developing identity, the potential for stress is very great.

Finally, the adolescent must face the possiblity of a commitment to work. Occupational identity is the fourth major area of stress. The young person must choose from several possibilities, reconciling beliefs and attitudes with the choice. The expansion of possibilities, while extending personal freedom, has also created a new set of stresses. A few generations ago it was probable that a coal miner's son would work in the mines, as well. Similarly, a young woman knew that unless she chose one of the few traditional female occupations, her alternative might be an early marriage. The new freedom has brought with it a different set of stresses, as work becomes equated with career. Seen as a way of life, one's work contributes powerfully to one's identity.

The idealism that is characteristic of young people may clash with economic realities. The fear of "selling out" haunts the young person on the verge of commitment. Some flee from commitment, avoiding the stress of decision making by prolonging school or dropping out. In extreme cases the lack of commitment may become a way of life, as an attempt is made to cope with the stress of decision making by avoidance. The successful resolution of the crisis of occupational choice results in a reconciliation, a harmonizing of inner values with reality demands.

Even under the best of circumstances, adolescence is stressful. It provides a graphic example of developmentally induced stress. The stresses of childhood and adolescence are an inevitable part of development, and they are necessary for growth. If they are prolonged and/or unusually severe, however, they can have damaging effects.

Endemic Social Stress

Unlike the specific instances of stress associated with discrete events and situations, there is a more general psychosocial stress endemic to society. In contemporary Western societies, the rapid social and technological changes of the past few decades have increasingly strained the capacity of individuals to adapt.

Children, like their parents, have had to cope with these social trends and the rapid changes they have spawned. While the implications of social change are beyond the scope of this book, one example might prove useful in elucidating how social change has affected parents and their children.

One major trend that emerged during the 1960s was embodied in the human potential movement. While the movement advocated the development of each human being's unique potential, it also provided a rationalization for selfishness. It fostered the myth that any number of potentials could be actualized in a process of growth without pain or sacrifice. However, when individuals sought to have all their own needs met, they often found it was at the expense of family and social responsibilities.

The precipitous rise in divorce rates, alternative living arrangements, and the general erosion of the family were some of the obvious changes encouraged by this trend. One important implication was found in the effect this trend had on parents' attitudes toward children.

In even the best of circumstances there is a natural ambivalence toward children. They require sacrifice, particularly on the mother's part, the postponing of personal goals and interests, restrictions on personal freedom and enjoyment, and economic burdens. Luckily, there are strong innate tendencies toward love and the protection of the young that counterbalance these feelings, so that children are assured a reasonable measure of parental love and acceptance.

However, when social trends exacerbate these ambivalent feelings, parents may be driven to increasingly extreme methods of coping. One extreme response may be found in instances when parents, in order to meet their own needs, foster a pseudo-maturity in children, often under the guise of encouraging independence. The children of those parents are essentially deprived of their childhood. Not allowed to be children, they are forced to try to cope with an adult reality for which they are not emotionally prepared.

Still another example of an extreme response may be found in instances when parents are tentative about accepting the responsibilities of parenthood. While occasionally they may openly abdicate that responsibility, it is more likely that they may hold back from a total commitment. The result is some withholding of love, or alternatively a giving and withholding, in an inconsistent pattern. The children of such parents react to what they perceive as a deprivation of parental love and they, in turn, may also adopt extreme behavior patterns in their efforts to cope with the resulting stress, confusion, and insecurity.

Anthony (1978) has pointed to the potentially disastrous consequences of this social trend:

> The growing disinterest in child rearing among young adults in our society and the trend toward the postponement of having children is increasingly evident. Not only are fewer children being produced in almost all the developed countries, but these are turned over to the care of others while parents go out to work. Some have seen this as questioning the existence of an innate drive toward parenthood . . . but it may well be that social and cultural factors have a much greater impact on our innate behavior than we hitherto realized. It may even be that in our child-rearing methods we are raising children who no longer care to raise children. I would thus agree with Rexford that one of the major risks to children of this century in the Western world . . . is the ambivalence of adults. This is a large psychological hammer hanging over the heads of children . . . (p. 13).

SUMMARY

Stress has been a fairly recent object of scientific inquiry, coming to the social sciences from biology. Initial studies were concerned with the effects of the emotions on bodily functions, and with the impact of traumatic events. Eventually, stress began to be seen in a broader psychosocial context. As the focus shifted, the definition of stress was broadened. Today, stress may be defined as a state of emotional tension arising from the failure of the environment to meet the individual's needs, and/or from events and situations that are seen as threatening.

There are many sources of stress, some of which are unique to childhood. The major sources of childhood stress are normal developmental stresses, endemic social stress, and specific traumatic events and situations.

REFERENCES

Achtenberg, J., Simonton, O., and Simonton, S. Stress, psychological factors and cancer. Fort Worth, Tex.: New Medicine Press, 1976.

Anthony, E. J. A new scientific region to explore. In E. J. Anthony and C. Koupernik (Eds.), The child in his family: Vulnerable children (Vol. 4). New York: Wiley, 1978.

Apply, M. H., and Trumbull, R. Psychological stress: Issues in research. New York: Appleton-Century-Crofts, 1967.

Arnold, M. Emotions and personality. New York: Columbia University Press, 1960.

Barrett, J. E. The relationship of life events to the onset of neurotic disorders. In J. E. Barrett (Ed.), Stress and mental disorder. New York: Raven Press, 1979.

Bettelheim, B. The informed heart: Autonomy in a mass age. Glencoe, Ill.: The Free Press, 1960.

Blaufarb, H., and Levine, J. Crisis intervention in an earthquake. Soc Work, July, 1972, 16-19.

Boike, M. F., Gesten, E. L., Cowen, E. L., Felner, R. D., and Francis, R. Relationship between family background problems and school problems and competencies of young normal children. Psychology in the Schools, 1978, 15, 283-290.

Brown, G. W. A three-factor causal model of depression. In J. E. Barrett (Ed.), Stress and mental disorder. New York: Raven Press, 1979.

Chandler, L. A. The source of stress inventory. Psychology in the Schools, 1981, 18, 164-168.

Cobb, S., and Rose, R. Hypertension, peptic ulcers, and diabetes in air traffic controllers. JAMA, 1973, 244, 489-492.

Coddington, R. D. The significance of life events and etiological factors in the diseases of children. J Psychosom Res, 1972, 16, 7-18.

Compton, A. Psychoanalytic theories. In I. L. Kutash et al. (Eds.), Handbook on stress and anxiety. San Francisco: Jossey-Bass, 1980.

Coyne, J. C., and Lazarus, R. S. Cognitive style, stress perception and coping. In I. L. Kutash et al. (Eds.), Handbook on stress and anxiety. San Francisco: Jossey-Bass, 1980.

Dohrenwend, B. P. Stressful life events and psychopathology: Some issues of theory and method. In J. E. Barrett (Ed.), Stress and mental disorder. New York: Raven Press, 1979.

Dohrenwend, B. S., and Dohrenwend, B. P. A brief historical introduction to research on stressful life events. In B. S. Dohrenwend and B. P. Dohrenwend (Eds.), Stressful life events: Their nature and effects. New York: Wiley, 1974.

Dohrenwend, B. S., Kransoff, L., Askenasy, A. R., and Dohrenwend, B. P. The Psychiatric Epidemiology Research Interview Life Events Scale. In L. Goldberger and S. Brenitz (Eds.), Handbook of stress: Theoretical and clinical aspects. New York: The Free Press, 1982.

Egeland, B., Schankel, J., Erikson, M. F., Rahe, D., and Mathieu, P. Development of social and emotional competence in high-risk preschool children. Paper presented at the annual meeting of the National Association of School Psychologists, Toronto, March, 1982.

Elkind, D. *Child development and education: A Piagetian perspective*. New York: Oxford University Press, 1976.

Endler, N. S. The case for person-situation interactions. *Can Psychological Rev*, 1975, *16*, 12-25.

Endler, N. S. Whence interactional psychology? In A. Furnham and M. Argyle (Eds.), *Social behavior in context*. Boston: Allyn and Bacon, 1982.

Endler, N. S., and Magnusson, D. Personality and person by situation interactions. In N. S. Endler and D. Magnusson (Eds.), *Interactional psychology and personality*. Washington, D.C.: Hemisphere, 1976.

Erikson, E. H. *Childhood and society*. New York: Norton, 1964.

Erikson, E. *Identity, youth and crisis*. New York: W. W. Norton & Co., 1968.

Farber, I. E. The role of motivation in verbal learning and performance. *Psychol Bull*, 1955, *52*, 311-327.

Felner, R. D., Ginter, M. A., Boike, M., and Cowen, E. L. Parental death or divorce and the school adjustment of young children. *American Journal of Community Psychology*, 1981, *9*, 181-190.

Felner, R. D., Stolberg, A., and Cowen, E. L. Crisis events and school mental health referral patterns of young children. *J Consult Clin Psychol*, 1975, *43*, 305-310.

Freud, A., and Burlingham, D. T. *War and children*. New York: Willard, 1943.

Freud, S. Beyond the pleasure principle (1928). *Standard Edition, 18*. London: Hogarth Press, 1962.

Garmezy, N. Children under stress: Perspectives on antecedents and correlates of vulnerability and resistance to psychopathology. In A. I. Rabin et al. (Eds.), Further explorations in personality. New York: Wiley, 1981.

Gersten, J. C., Langner, T. S., Eisenberg, J. C., and Orzeck, L. Child behavior and life events: Undesirable change or change per se? In B. S. Dohrenwend and B. P. Dohrenwend (Eds.), Stressful life events: Their nature and effects. New York: Wiley, 1974.

Gersten, J. C., Langner, T. S., Eisenberg, J. G., and Simcha-Fagan, O. An evaluation of the etiologic role of stressful life-change events in psychological disorders. J Health Soc Behav, 1977, 18, 228-244.

Gesten, E. L., Sher, K., and Cowen, E. L. Judged school problems and competencies of referred children with varying family background characteristics. J Abnorm Child Psychol, 1978, 6, 247-255.

Goffman, E. The presentation of self in everyday life. Garden City, N.Y.: Doubleday, 1959.

Grinker, K., and Spiegel, S. Men under stress. Philadelphia: Blakiston, 1945.

Haan, N. The assessment of coping, defense and stress. In L. Goldberger and S. Breznitz (Eds.), Handbook of stress: Theoretical and clinical aspects. New York: The Free Press, 1982.

Heisel, J. S., Ream, S., Raitz, R., Rappaport, M., and Coddington, R. D. The significance of life events as contributing factors in the diseases of children. J Pediatr, 1973, 83, 199-123.

Hoesch, A. H. Stressful life events of children: Their incidence, magnitude and classification. Unpublished doctoral dissertation. University of Pittsburgh, 1983.

Holmes, T. H. Development and application of a quantitative measure of life change magnitude. In J. E. Barrett (Ed.), Stress and mental disorder. New York: Raven Press, 1979.

Holmes, T. H., and Masuda, M. Life change and illness susceptibility. In B. S. Dohrenwend and B. P. Dohrenwend (Eds.), _Stressful life events: Their nature and effects_. New York: Wiley, 1974.

Holmes, T. H., and Rahe, R. H. The Social Readjustment Rating Scale. _J Psychosom Res_, 1967, _11_, 213-218.

Horowitz, M., Schaefer, C., and Cooney, P. Life event scoring for recency of experience. In E. K. Gunderson and R. H. Rahe (Eds.), _Life stress and illness_. Springfield, Ill.: Charles Thomas Co., 1974.

Hurst, M. W. Life changes and psychiatric symptom development: Issues of content, scoring and clustering. In J. E. Barrett (Ed.), _Stress and mental disorders_. New York: Raven Press, 1979.

Jacobsen, F. _Progressive relaxation_. Chicago: University of Chicago Press, 1938.

James, W. _Some problems in philosophy_. New York: Longmans Green and Co., 1911.

Janis, I. L. Psychological effects of warning. In D. Chapman and G. Baker (Eds.), _Man and society in disaster_. New York: Basic Books, 1962.

Kaplan, H. B. Sociological theories. In L. Kutash et al. _Handbook on stress and anxiety_. San Francisco, Calif.: Jossey-Bass, 1980.

Kardiner, A., and Spiegel, H. _War stress and neurotic illness_. New York: Hoeber, 1947.

Kessler, J. _Psychopathology of childhood_. Englewood Cliffs, N.J.: Prentice-Hall, 1966.

Kinston, W., and Rosser, R. Disaster: Effects on mental and physical state. _J Psychosom Res_, 1974, _18_, 437-456.

Langer, T. S., and Michael, S. T. _Life stress and mental health_. London: Oxford University Press, 1963.

Lazarus, R. S. _Patterns of adjustment_. New York: McGraw-Hill, 1976.

Lazarus, R. S., and Launier, R. Stress-related transactions between person and environment. In L. A. Previn and M. Lewis (Eds.), Perspectives in interactional psychology. New York: Plenum, 1978.

Lerner, M. In S. Cunningham. Stress research moves from lab to workplace. APA Monitor, 1982, 13 (6), 19.

Lewin, K. A dynamic theory of personality. New York: McGraw-Hill, 1935.

Lief, A. The commonsense psychiatry of Dr. Adolf Meyer. New York: McGraw-Hill, 1948.

Lorimor, R. J., Justice, B., McBee, G. W., and Weinman, M. Weighting events in life-events research. J Health Soc Behav, 1979, 20, 306-308.

Maddi, S. Personality theories: A comparative analysis. Homewood, Ill.: Dorsey Press, 1968.

Magnusson, D. Situational determinants of stress: An interactional perspective. In L. Goldberger and S. Breznitz (Eds.), Handbook of stress: Theoretical and clinical aspects. New York: The Free Press, 1982.

Maslow, A. H. Motivation and personality. New York: Harper, 1954.

McGrath, J. E. A conceptual formulation for research on stress. In J. E. McGrath (Ed.), Social and psychological factors in stress. New York: Holt, Rinehart and Winston, 1970.

Miller, N. E. Learning of visceral and glandular responses. Science, 1969, 163, 434-445.

Moore, T. W. Studying the growth of personality. Vita Humanitatis, 1959, 2, 65-87.

Moore, T. W., Hindley, C. B., and Falkner, F. A. A longitudinal research in child development and some of its problems. Br Med J, 1954, 2, 1123-1137.

Mulvey, M. A. The relationship of life events, gender and age: A community study of adulthood. Unpublished doctoral dissertation, City University of New York, 1979.

Murphy, G. Affect and perceptual learning. Psychol Rev, 1956, 3, 1-15.

Murray, H. A. Explorations in personality. New York: Oxford University Press, 1938.

Mutter, A. Z., and Schliefer, N. J. The role of psychological and social factors in the onset of somatic illness in children. Psychosom Med, 1966, 28, 333-343.

Newman, J. Children of disaster: Clinical observations at Buffalo Creek. Am J Psychiatry, 1976, 133, 306-312.

Paykel, E. S. Life events and acute depression. In J. P. Scott and E. C. Senway (Eds.), Separation and depression: Clinical and research aspects. Washington, D.C.: AAAS, 1973.

Paykel, E. S., Prusoff, B. A., and Uhlenhuth, E. H. Scaling of life events. Arch Gen Psychiatry, 1971, 25, 340-347.

Paykel, E. S., and Uhlenhuth, E. H. Rating the magnitude of life events. Can Psychiatr Assoc J, 1972, 17, 93-100.

Piaget, J. Play, dreams and imitation in childhood. New York: Norton, 1951.

Rahe, R. H., and Arthur, R. J. Life change and illness studies: Past history and future directions. J Human Stress, 1978, 4, 3-15.

Rahe, R. H., and Lind, E. Psychosocial factors and sudden cardiac death: A pilot study. J Psychosom Res, 1971, 15, 19-24.

Rahe, R. H., and Paasikivi, J. Psychosocial factors and myocardial infarction. II: An outpatient study in Sweden. J Psychosom Res, 1971, 15, 33-39.

Rolf, J. E., and Garmezy, N. The school performance of children vulnerable to behavior pathology. In D. F. Ricks et al. (Eds.), Life history research in psychopathology (Vol. 3). Minneapolis, Minn.: University of Minnesota Press, 1974.

Ruitenbeek, H. M. Varieties of personality theory. New York: Dutton, 1964.

Sandler, I. N. Social support resources, stress and maladjustment of poor children. Am J Community Psychol, 1980, 8, 41-52.

Sandler, I. N., and Block, M. Life stress and maladaptation of children. Am J Community Psychol, 1979, 7, 425-440.

Sandler, I. N., and Ramsey, T. B. Dimensional analysis of children's stressful life events. Am J Community Psychol, 1980, 8, 285-302.

Sarason, I. G., and Sarason, B. R. The importance of cognition and moderator variables in stress. In D. Magnusson (Ed.), Towards a psychology of situations: An interactional perspective. Hillsdale, N.Y.: Erlbaum, 1981.

Selye, H. The stress of life. New York: McGraw-Hill, 1956.

Siegal, D. J. Separation-loss events, self concept, locus of control, and children's effective functioning in school. Unpublished doctoral dissertation, University of Pittsburgh, 1981.

Silber, E., Perry, S. E., and Bloch, D. A. Patterns of parent-child interaction in a disaster. Am J Psychiatry, 1957, 21, 159-167.

Stoyva, J., and Anderson, C. A coping-rest model of relaxation and stress management. In L. Goldberger and S. Breznitz (Eds.), Handbook of stress: Theoretical and clinical aspects. New York: The Free Press, 1982.

Tolman, E. C. Purposive behavior in animals and men. New York: 1932.

Wheatley, L. Stress and the heart. New York: Raven Press, 1981.

3

THE EFFECTS OF STRESS

The individual's experience of stress is a complex physiological, psychosocial, and behavioral phenomenon. In some cases psychological dysfunctions have been found to have physical effects. In other cases, physical disorders have caused psychological upset. Then there are those instances when the two types of problems may be so enmeshed, each exacerbating the other, that a primary condition cannot be clearly identified.

There is a voluminous amount of research literature on the study of stress, much of it devoted to the relationship between the physical and the psychological (compare, Selye, 1976). A comprehensive review of this literature would be beyond the scope of this book. However, a brief overview might be useful to gain some understanding of the impact of stress.

PSYCHOPHYSIOLOGICAL REACTIONS TO STRESS

While the psychological experience may be described as a state of emotional tension, its physical analogue is a state of nervous system arousal. The part of the nervous system most involved is the autonomic nervous system. Normally responsible for regulating those essential bodily functions usually seen as outside of conscious control, such as heart beat, breathing, and digestion, this system has a special role in preparing the individual for action in response to threat.

The stress reaction is seen as a defense to environmental threat. A stimulus is first received by the cortex through the sensory organs, and interpreted there as one of threat. The physiologic reaction is triggered by the pathways of the cerebral cortex, the brain's reticular activating system, and the release of substances that activate the pituitary and hypothalamus glands.

The pituitary gland, located below the brain, has been called the master gland, since it regulates the activities of the other glands. It releases a variety of hormones that influence growth and development, and it has a specific role in stress situations. In a stress reaction the pituitary releases adrenocorticotropic hormone (ACTH) which stimulates the adrenal glands to secrete the corticoids. These hormones influence other parts of the body in the stress reaction. As hormonal levels rise in the blood, sensors are activated that control the further release of hormones, in a complex feedback loop.

The hypothalamic-pituitary-adrenal axis plays the major role in the organism's efforts to cope with various threats. The adrenal glands produce two corticoids of particular importance in a stress reaction. They are the catecholamines: epinephrine and norepinephrine. Epinephrine makes the heart beat faster and seems to be released when the individual is afraid. Norepinephrine constricts the blood vessels, thereby raising the blood pressure. It seems to be released when an individual experiences anger. Norepinephrine is also carried back to the pituitary where it triggers the release of more ACTH, which then stimulates the adrenals to increase the rate of metabolism of carbohydrates, making the body's tissue generally more tense. Through the release of neurohormones and endocrine hormones the necessary changes in autonomic functions are affected to prepare the individual for fight or flight.

The stress reaction includes a rise in the rate of heartbeat and blood pressure. The blood vessels leading to the heart dilate, as do the bronchioles leading to the lungs, which serves to increase the oxygenation of the blood. Blood circulation is directed away from the skin and digestive system, allowing more blood to be directed toward the skeletal muscles. There is an increase in muscle tone and sweating. Cell metabolism slows to save energy, while stored glycogen is returned to provide more sugar for extra energy. The pupils of the eyes widen to permit more light to enter. The individual is prepared to respond to the threat.

Endocrine, cardiovascular, and related changes that occur in stress situations can be measured as indicators of the strength of the physiologic reaction. Selye (1976) has provided an extensive review of many of the studies employing physiologic measures. A few selected studies employing such methods might be useful as illustrations of this line of research.

Rose, Hurst, and Herd (1979), in a major study, followed 400 air traffic controllers over a three-year period. Psychiatric status, changes in affect, heart rate, blood pressure, and hormonal changes taken from blood samples, were carefully studied during that period. They found that individuals who showed increased blood pressure, cortisol, or growth-hormone levels in response to work were not at increased risk for psychiatric or psychological problems. They concluded that cardiovascular and endocrine responses to work were not associated with psychological problems, although such responses were predictors of various physical ailments.

The excretion rates of certain byproducts of the corticoids can be measured in plasma and urine samples taken from subjects in stress situations. This provides a measure of the strength of the reaction, so that the influence of mediating factors can be studied. An example of a typical study along this line was provided by Wolff et al. (1964) in their observations of a group of parents whose children were dying of leukemia. They were interested in finding out how a subject's psychological defenses might influence their psychophysiological reactions.

Throughout this stressful experience, they periodically measured the parents' excretion of 17-hydroxycorticosteroid (17-OHCS). Some parents handled the stress successfully by repression, and by gaining some distance by projecting their concerns onto cancer victims in general. These parents continued to show normal 17-OHCS excretion rates. On the other hand, those parents who were less successful in coping, admitting to feelings of despair, showed abnormally elevated 17-OHCS excretion rates.

This method has been used extensively in stress research with numerous populations in various settings to study individual differences and other mediating factors that influence the effects of stress. These individual differences are likely to be especially important in determining the predisposition to certain psychomatic disorders.

Psychosomatic Effects

Bodily damage can result when stress reactions are prolonged and/or severe. Duncan (1983) has described two general effects on children's health. First, stress reactions can directly damage tissues, especially those of the circulatory system. Since the reaction raises blood pressure, additional strain is placed on the heart, kidneys, and blood vessels. These effects, however, are usually gradual, and have little immediate effect on the heart. The second effect has to do with the body's immune system. Adrenal hormones reduce the ability of lymphocytes to recognize foreign bodies, and to produce antibodies to assist in fighting disease. The stress reaction, by increasing the amount of adrenal hormones, serves to suppress the immune system, thus reducing the body's defenses to disease.

Duncan sees these effects as the reason why children who have experienced more stressful life events are more likely to be susceptible to illness. He cites studies of strep bacterial infection in children which found that 30 percent of all well children had the infection present in their throats, although they showed no symptoms of the illness. When the majority of children with the infection who did not have the symptoms were compared with a minority who did, it was found that one fourth of the children's sore throats followed a family crisis. An ill child was four times as likely to have just experienced a stressful life event as one of the infected but healthy children.

This increased susceptibility may help to explain the findings of greater environmental stress among children hospitalized for developmental and psychophysiologic disorders (Beitchman and Dielman, 1982).

In addition to the general effects on children's health, psychophysiological reactions may selectively but severely impair certain aspects of body functioning. The resulting problems, traditionally seen as psychosomatic, that is psychogenic in origin, may contain particular configurations of physiological and emotional (including psychodynamic family) components (Gottschalk, 1983). A discussion of some of the more common psychosomatic disorders may help better to define these configurations.

Asthma

It has been estimated that one out of every five children has some type of allergic reaction (for example, asthma, eczema, hay fever, and so on) (Rappaport, Howard, and Flint, 1976). One of the most common childhood reactions is asthma. The symptoms of asthma include difficulty in inspiring and expiring air, sensations of chest tightening, and characteristic wheezing during the expiratory phase of breathing. It is brought about by episodic narrowing of the air passages from the windpipe to the lungs. The asthma attack occurs as a reflex reaction to local irritation of the bronchial tissue, or as a result of direct innervation from the hypothalamus during emotional arousal. It is found in about 2 percent of the child population, and is more common in boys than in girls (Graham et al., 1967; Purcell, 1975).

Asthmatic attacks may be caused by three factors, alone or in combination: (1) exceptional sensitivity of the bronchial tissue to allergens, substances that produce allergic reactions; (2) infection, such as pneumonia; and/or (3) emotional factors. It has been estimated that approximately half of the asthma cases can be attributed to some combination of allergic, infective, and emotional factors (Rees, 1963).

It is often argued that asthmatic children, like many with psychosomatic complaints, do not represent a homogeneous group. Rather such children may differ widely in terms of their psychological and physiological makeup and the etiology of their problems, although they share a similar set of symptoms. Therefore, in studying asthma many investigators have seen the need to divide the asthmatic group into more meaningful subgroups.

One important distinction has been suggested by Bernstein and Purcell (1963). They found that some children quickly lost their asthmatic symptoms after being hospitalized away from their families, while other children showed no improvement and required continuous steroid treatment. This suggested that, for at least some of the asthmatics, the parent-child relationship might be an important precipitating factor. In order to rule out other home environmental factors as precipitants, Purcell et al. (1969) conducted a later experiment in which they followed two groups of asthmatic children, those with a history of asthmatic attacks preceded by emotional arousal, and those without such a history. After establishing baseline rates for the symptoms, the family was temporarily moved out of the home while the child stayed in the home with an adult caretaker. After two weeks the families were reunited. Those children who had a history of emotional arousal prior to attacks showed considerable improvement during the separation, while the other children showed little change during the same period.

A useful measure, sensitive to the two broad categories of asthmatic children, is the Allergy Potential Scale (APS). This instrument assesses the incidence of allergies in the child's family, a blood count, a skin test for reactivity to allergies, the total number of allergies, and the ease of diagnosing certain allergies. It can be used as an indicator of the child's somatic predisposition to asthma. Children scoring high on the APS presumably would be those with a greater constitutional susceptibility to asthma, while those scoring low would have lower physiological predisposition to the disorder.

Block and colleagues (Block et al., 1964; Block, 1968) studied the characteristics of children and their parents by dividing an asthmatic group into high scorers and low scorers on the APS. They found that low scorers showed significantly more emotional immaturity than high scorers. In addition, their mothers showed more unhealthy attitudes, including overprotection and ambivalence toward motherhood.

While there is evidence of parental, and especially maternal behavior and attitudes playing a part in the development of asthma (Block et al., 1964; Rees, 1963), the exact nature of that relationship has not been shown.

Sperling (1968) has formulated a psychodynamic hypothesis based on her observations of asthmatic children. She refers to the interaction as a psychosomatic relationship between mother and child, which may precipitate the onset of asthma in a child who is constitutionally predisposed. Sperling sees the child as being rejected when he is healthy and striving toward independence. On the other hand, when he is sick and dependent, he is reinforced by maternal attention. The child's illness is then in response to the mother's need to control and keep her child dependent on her. Since the aggressive feelings which the child experiences in this situation cannot be expressed overtly, they find expression in the asthmatic symptoms.

In an effort to test the relative contribution of psychogenic and biologic factors in allergies, Jacobs et al. (1967) have hypothesized a summation model, which holds that both factors would be present to a moderate degree in allergic reactions. Using a technique similar to Block's, they derived an additive score for several physiologic measures as an index of biologic predisposition. Psychologic predisposition was seen in terms of prior faulty family experiences that resulted in exaggerated dependency of the child on a dominating mother. Because of his background, such life situations as separation from or loss of maternal control and protection are perceived by the child as threatening and potentially disabling. At that point when previously appropriate passive, submissive modes fail to continue to secure maternal reinforcement and the loss of maternal domination is present, illness develops.

Various psychological measures were employed to assess aspects of the mother-child relationship as hypothesized by the investigators. In a study of 65 male college students, they found that 75.6 percent of the cases of allergic illness showed both biologic and psychologic factors present, supporting the summation model. In addition, considerable support was found for their hypothesized parent-child relationship.

Enuresis

Enuresis is the term used for the lack of appropriate control in the elimination of urine. Estimates of prevalence vary, as does the meaning of "appropriate control." Both the age of the child and the frequency of incidents are variables to consider in defining the condition. Generally, bladder control is achieved by four years of age, but occasional bedwetting by older children is not unusual, and may or may not be seen as a problem.

Lapouse and Monk (1959) reported that 8 percent of the school-age children in their sample wet the bed at least once a month, while Rutter, Yule, and Graham (1973) have reported nocturnal enuresis in 20 to 25 percent of the child population. After age five enuresis is more severe and more common in boys than in girls (Oppel, Harper, and Rowland, 1968).

There is a wide range of opinion regarding etiology of enuresis. Psychodynamic theorists, learning theorists, and physicians have all speculated as to its probable cause (Lovibond and Coote, 1969).

From the behavioral perspective, enuresis results from a failure in learning. This may be due to faulty toilet training, or to the disruptive influence of anxiety on the learning process. In any case, it is a control response that has not been acquired.

Psychodynamic theorists see enuresis as a symptom of some underlying emotional disorder. Achenbach and Lewis (1971) provide an example of a psychodynamic family explanation. As with the other psychosomatic disorders, they see the personalities of the parents as important contributing factors. They theorize that both parents, because of their own needs, tend to emasculate the enuretic boy, and so the boy begins to see his masculinity as a threat. As a consequence, the child adopts a passive orientation, relinquishing responsibility for his body to others and failing to achieve mastery. They tested some of these speculations with a group of boys seen for outpatient services at the Yale Child Study Center. Consistent with their hypotheses, they found that mothers of enuretics were more masculine and tended to emasculate their sons more than the mothers of a similar group referred for learning disabilities.

Physicians have also speculated about dysfunctions of the urinary tract or nervous system, which may be causative factors. Obstructive lesions and defects of the adrenergic mechanisms that cause bladder tightening have also been suspected as contributing factors (Mahoney, 1971). A possible genetic-constitutional predisposition in some cases is suggested by the findings of an increased incidence of enuresis within families (Bakwin, 1961).

In a recent study of enureses of various origins, Trombini et al. (1982) analyzed the movement of the bladder muscle in a group of children with nocturnal enuresis under conditions of experimentally induced stress. They found that muscle contraction was present in a subgroup of children with psychogenic enuresis, but absent in those whose problems were caused by organic lesions. Moreover, the motor response increased as the level of emotional tension increased.

Further evidence for the association of enuresis with stress comes from the findings of family disruption and disorganization, such as broken homes, mother-child separation, and maternal incompetence in the histories of enuretics (Oppel et al., 1968; Stein and Susser, 1966, 1967).

Nevertheless, there are those who contend that enuresis is not inevitably associated with emotional disturbance. Werry (1979), after reviewing a number of studies, concluded that there was a small but significant correlation between enuresis and psychopathology. However, he pointed out that most of the studies employed clinic-referred samples, and he implied that the majority of enuretics in the general population would not show emotional disturbance. Moreover, in those who do, the relationship between enuresis and emotional problems is unclear.

Anorexia Nervosa

Anorexia may be defined as food refusal accompanied by an intense fear of becoming obese, which results in extreme weight loss. While once thought to be rather rare, there is evidence that it is becoming an increasing problem. The disorder occurs predominantly in females. It has been estimated that as many as one in 250 females between 12 to 18 years of age may develop the disorder (APA, 1980). The most frequent age of onset is between 17 and 18 years of age (Crisp, 1980).

The central feature of anorexia nervosa is the adolescent's marked pursuit of thinness with the associated conviction that her body is too large. Garfinkle and Garner (1982), in their excellent review of the condition, describe the typical course of events:

> The initial intent is to "lose a few pounds" . . . However, when her weight goal has been attained, she still feels somewhat overweight and then gradually decides to further restrict her intake of foods. Usually this takes place over several months and goes unnoticed by those around her. . . . The drive for thinness is egosyntonic, and is not viewed as something they would like to see changed. They don't perceive themselves as abnormal.

Anorexia has been studied from a number of perspectives including the individual's psychological characteristics, the physiological functions, family dynamics, and social-cultural aspects.

A psychophysiological understanding of this disorder continues to be elusive. One of the confounding factors is that much of the research has been done on women who have been identified as anorexic and therefore it is difficult to know if the physiological changes which may differentiate them from control groups are predisposing to, or the result of, the anorexic condition. Garfinkle and Garner (1983) address this issue by noting that there is considerable evidence of hypothalamic dysfunction in anorexic patients. Many of the manifestations of that dysfunction, however, can be attributed to the weight loss or caloric restrictions, while others may in part reflect emotional distress. They suggest that hypothalamic dysfunctions may contribute to the self-perpetuating aspect of the disorder.

Many of the psychological studies of anorexia have followed suggestions advanced by the psychoanalytic approach to the disorder. Psychoanalytic theorists have seen it as a failure in separation-individuation in the mother-daughter relationship (Bruch, 1978; Goetz, 1977; Ehrensing and Weitzman, 1970; Hamilton, 1975). In their formulations the growing child's needs are routinely subverted to the mother's sense of what is appropriate. The result is that the anorexic child does not develop a consistent, differentiated sense of self. She does not discriminate her needs from her parents', becoming a devoted compliant child with little capacity for autonomous functioning. Bruch (1978) sees this compliant mode as being functional until adolescence with its normal demands for separation and individuation. The adolescent identity crisis, then, becomes an important component in the genesis of anorexia.

Bruch (1973) sees the parents of the anorexic as overconcerned and ambitious. They expect and reward obedience and performance. As long as the child complies, all is well, but the child's growing need for independence as adolescence approaches is not accepted by the parents. From this perspective, the basic issue is a fear of not being in control. The struggle for control with the parents takes on pathological dimensions. It is expressed in dependency on the home, open rejection of everything from the parents, and the inability to make decisions.

Recently, there has been interest in a more extended analysis of the family such as that offered by the family systems approach (Minuchin et al., 1978; Selvini-Palazzoli, 1978). Minuchin and associates have described the anorexic's family as having an enmeshed, undifferentiated quality, characterized by weak boundaries between individuals. The primary concern is the maintenance of overt harmony and closeness. Loyalty, self-sacrifice, and the anticipation of the needs of others are highly valued, while disagreement and conflict are seen as threats to family cohesion. Generational boundaries may be poorly defined with a parent acting like a rivalrous sibling or allowing the child to assume the role of parent or spouse. This may result in any number of unusual alliances, with the child encouraged to side with one parent against the other. Other characteristics of such families include overinvolvement, overprotectiveness, rigidity, and a lack of conflict resolution (Minuchin et al., 1978).

In discussing the role of family interrelationships in the genesis of the disorder, Garfinkle and Garner (1982) conclude that there is no single type of mother-daughter relationship regularly associated with anorexia nervosa. Moreover, they do not feel that the disorder is always related to major problems in the mother-daughter relationship. Rather, they maintain that there are a variety of familial relationships that may be important.

Gastrointestinal Ulceration

The association between ulcers and stress has been frequently commented upon in the professional and popular literature. There are three types of gastrointestinal ulceration: (1) peptic ulcers, which are lesions of the stomach; (2) duodenal ulcers, which are lesions in the lining of the duodenum, the top section of the small intestine; and (3) ulcerative colitis, which are lesions in the large intestine.

Ulcers are formed by an excess of acid secretion in the stomach which eventually eats away the linings of the stomach or duodenum, forming the ulcer. Stomach acidity has been shown to increase under conditions of environmental stress by means of the hypothalamic-pituitary-adrenal axis. However, while stress stimulates stomach secretions, it causes ulceration only in predisposed individuals (Selye, 1976).

The cause of ulcerative colitis is unknown, although because of the wide range of systemic complaints, an immunologic basis is frequently postulated (Finch and Hansen, 1980). The major symptoms of colitis are pain, diarrhea, and bleeding from the intestinal tract. Both conditions have been found to be associated with stressful situations, and there is ample evidence to suggest that children are at least as much subject to ulcer formation as are adults (Selye, 1976).

In a recent investigation designed to study the personalities of ulcer patients, Lyketsos et al. (1982) compared a group of patients with hypertensive patients, patients hospitalized for other (nonpsychosomatic) complaints, and a control group. These investigators were looking for personality characteristics that might be consistent with the psychoanalytic view, as explicated by Alexander (1950), which held that such patients should show dependency needs. They found evidence of low dominance and excessive dependence in the two psychosomatic groups, suggesting some support for the psychoanalytic view of such individuals as those who choose to handle aggression and hostile tendencies, which are viewed as unacceptable by the individual, by lowered dominance and increased dependency.

One major difficulty confounding research that seeks to associate personality characteristics with psychosomatic disorders has been commented on above. It is the problem of trying to determine if the personality manifestations are predisposing to, or the effects of, the physical symptoms.

Sandberg and Bliding (1975) commented on this problem. They criticized most experimental studies of ulcer disorders by pointing out that, in most studies, the experimental group is selected because they already show ulcer symptoms. This confounds the problem since it may well be that emotional factors are the result of the ulcers, and not causative factors. They reasoned, therefore, that it would be best to use an unselected group. They chose to study an unselected group of army trainees. Upon analyzing the data from a series of measures administered as they went through basic training, the investigators found that those who developed ulcers did not differ significantly from other trainees on psychological measures. All had undergone the same stress experiences associated with the training, but some tended to react with gastrointestinal symptoms. The group that contracted duodenal ulcers during basic training was found to be very heterogeneous regarding personality and triggering problems, and to be quite similar to all other trainees.

In summing up the physiological/psychological issue with ulcerative colitis, Davidson and Silverberg (1982) probably came close to the most widely accepted position that can be applied to the psychosomatic disorders in general. They begin by stating that the physiological component may be seen as an infectious process and hence the immune system is suspected. They go on to discuss the psychological component, and they point out that, as with other psychosomatic disorders, many patients are passive, rigid, and oversensitive, with an excessive need for love, and with mothers who are demanding, cold, and punitive. However, they maintain that not all patients or all mothers share these characteristics, and these features are probably not of primary importance. They conclude with a statement that may have relevance for many of the psychosomatic disorders:

> It is likely that there are multiple determinants including personality patterns of both mother and child as well as environmental influences such as separation phenomena. Whatever emotional factors are important, there is little doubt that once the disease is established, exacerbations and remissions are often associated with changes in emotional state.

PSYCHOLOGICAL AND BEHAVIORAL EFFECTS

Effects on School, Family, and Social Functioning

The effects of stress, particularly if it is prolonged and severe, can be pervasive. We have already seen its effects on physical functioning, and it may affect other major areas of functioning as well. Freud's famous dictum that a problem is significant when it affects the individual's ability to love or work calls attention to two essential aspects of human experience. For the child, work is equated with school performance, for it is in school that one's resources must be marshalled for sustained, concentrated, and goal-oriented effort. Love, in the broadest sense, encompasses the range of family and social relations, including the capacity for positive interpersonal bonds.

The adverse influence of stress on general school functioning and academic performance has been clearly demonstrated (Felner, Ginter, Boike, and Cowen, 1981; Felner, Stolberg, and Cowen, 1975; Gesten, Scher, and

Cowen, 1978; Mullins et al., 1982; Sandler and Block, 1979; Shinn, 1978; Siegel, 1981). A brief review of a few of the relevant studies may provide a better understanding of that impact.

Shinn (1978) conducted an extensive review of the literature on the detrimental effects of father absence on children's cognitive development as assessed by standardized IQ and achievement tests, and school performance. She found that in single-parent families financial hardship, high levels of anxiety, and low levels of parent-child interaction were all associated with poor school performance by children.

Felner et al. (1975) studied two types of stressful experiences found in the histories of primary grade school children: parental death and divorce. Both "crisis" groups were compared, first to demographically matched referred controls without crisis histories, and then to each other. Teachers were asked to rate the children with reference to the amount of maladjustment they showed in school by using the AML, a screening instrument, and the Teacher Referral Form. Each experimental group had a significantly higher overall maladjustment score than its comparable control group. Children with a history of parental death were significantly more anxious, depressed, and withdrawn than the matched controls, whereas separation/divorced children had more aggressive and acting-out problems than their controls.

In a subsequent study, Felner et al. (1981) further examined the effects of parental divorce or death on the school adjustment of young children. Children with a history of these stressful life events were found to show greater overall school maladaptation than children without such histories. Children of divorce had significantly more acting-out problems, and those with histories of parental death had more shy-anxious problems than their control groups. The authors concluded that the association between specific crisis history and specific school adjustment patterns may have implications for the study of coping with stressful life events and for preventive efforts.

Sandler and Block (1979) extended the investigation of children under stress beyond the school to include the home. They asked teachers to identify maladapting children in four inner city schools. Teachers then rated the maladaptive and control children on dimensions of maladaptive behavior using the AML screening instrument. Four scores were derived: A (acting out), M (moody-withdrawn), L (learning problems), and a summative score AML. Parents were also asked to rate their children's behavior using selected items derived from the Louisville Behavior Checklist. Items selected were from the factor-analyzed derived dimensions of the scale: sensitivity, social withdrawal, fear, infantile aggression, antisocial, hyperactivity, and two content scores: prosocial and academic ability. They then compared the children's recent life histories by using a life events schedule modified from Coddington's scale for elementary school children.

In their analysis of the data the investigators found that one of the demographic variables, source of income (on welfare), also differentiated the maladjusted from the control group. Therefore, they further divided the maladapting group into two subgroups, those whose families were on welfare and those whose families were not. In general, maladapting children were more likely to have been on welfare, and to have experienced significantly more stressful life events during the previous year, than the matched control group. When the maladapting group was divided into welfare and nonwelfare subgroups, it was found that the nonwelfare maladapting group had experienced more life events than either the nonwelfare controls or the maladapting welfare children. Moreover, the nonwelfare maladapting group showed a high correlation of parent ratings of behavior problems with the measures of life events.

In a study that went beyond the school and family to examine the broader issue of the effects of stress on social relations, Hetherington (1972) studied the effects of father absence due to divorce or death on adolescent girls. She found disruptions in their interactions with males. With daughters of divorce this behavior took the form of proximity seeking with males, early heterosexual behavior, and more open responsiveness. In contrast, the daughters of widows showed inhibition, rigidity, avoidance, and restraint around males.

Further information on the psychological effects of stress can be gained by studying the emotional reactions of children in those extreme stress situations found in the literature on disasters. As has been pointed out in Chapter 2, a number of studies of children in disaster situations have shown similar results in the pattern of the child's psychological responses. Irrational fears, confusion, anxiety and feelings of helplessness as well as regression and an increase in dependency behavior have commonly been reported (Blaufarb and Levine, 1972; Newman, 1976; Silber, Perry, and Bloch, 1957).

In sum, stress has been found to be associated with poor school performance, ineffective functioning at school and in the home, problems in social relations, and a variety of emotional reactions. In order to gain a better appreciation of the impact of stressful experiences on children, let us now focus on three examples:

Death of a Parent

The loss of a loved one is always a painful experience. The nature and severity of the effects of stress on the child who has lost a parent through death will vary depending on a number of mediating factors.

The most common reaction seems to include initial incidents of acting out or conduct disorders, usually following, or within a few months of, the loss (Epstein, Weitz, Roback, and McKee, 1975). This initial reaction is followed by lowered self-esteem, guilt, and depression (Grossberg and Crandell, 1978). Other behavior disorders have been associated with parental loss such as depressive and phobic disorders, and school refusal (Arthur and Kemme, 1964; Caplan and Douglas, 1969, Black, 1974). Some maintain that the effects may not be seen for months or even years. Rutter (1966), for example, found that in his clinic sample there was a gap of five years or more between parental death and the onset of symptoms in the child.

In general, the studies have shown that the loss of a parent by death is a stressful event for a child, and one that may be associated with impaired emotional development and/or psychopathology (Bendikson and Fulton, 1975; Epstein et al., 1975; Markusen and Fulton, 1971; Shepherd and Barraclough, 1976). For example, Kirkpatrick, Samuels, Jones, and Zweibelson (1965) found that children who experienced the loss of a parent through death showed reduced academic achievement, more physical illness and psychological adjustment reactions. Lifschitz (1976) reported that bereaved children displayed greater oppositional behavior, restlessness, and restriction of general cognitive level when compared to a matched control group.

Age has been shown to be an important factor influencing the effects of stress in this situation, as have the sex and ordinal position of the child. Children most at risk are those who have lost a parent during the ages of three to five years, or in early adolescence (Black, 1978). Being the oldest sibling seems to increase the risk, while having an older sibling of the same sex as the dead parent apparently protects against subsequent disorder (Birtchnell, 1971). Still another important mediating factor concerns the support provided by the surviving parent. The surviving parent's response, efforts to cope, availability, and the support he or she can provide in this stressful situation have been found to be of considerable importance in mitigating the effects of stress (Pattison, 1976; Silverman and Silverman, 1979).

While the death of a parent can be seen to cause some emotional adjustment difficulties, the association is not inevitable. While the event is always stressful, some children can cope more effectively than others. The evidence suggests that the majority of bereaved children never come to professional attention. Birtchnell (1971), for example, found that about 10 percent of his inpatient sample had lost a parent before the age of five years, while in a control group the incidence rate was 5 percent. Like other major life events, the loss of a parent by death can be seen as a crisis or a relatively mild stressful event depending on the child's personality, coping resources, circumstances, and the responses of significant adults.

Divorce

While divorce is often seen as a major stressful event, it is more accurate to view it as a stress situation, since it may involve weeks, months, or even years of varying degrees of family disruption and turmoil. Hetherington (1979) recognized that point when she advocated that we view divorce as

> a sequence of experiences involving a transition in the lives of children. This transition involves a shift from the family situation before the divorce to the disequilibrium and disorganization associated with separation and divorce, through a period when family members are experimenting with a variety of coping mechanisms. . . . This is followed by the reorganization and even-

> tual attainment of a new pattern of equilibrium in a single-parent household (p. 851).

Divorce causes considerable disruption in the life of the child, even in those situations where the parents may separate on more or less amicable terms. Family moves and relocations, changes in financial support, different child-care arrangements, and possibly a change of school and friends all may accompany the divorce and act as additional sources of stress with which the child may have to cope.

Like the other stress experiences, the effects of divorce are influenced by a variety of mediators including the psychological characteristics of the child, parental attitudes and behavior, and social supports. In addition, important differences have been found between the sexes and among various age groups.

The impact of divorce has been found to be more pervasive and enduring for boys than for girls. They show a higher rate of behavior disorders and problems in interpersonal relations in home and in school with teachers and peers. Both boys and girls also show increases in dependent and attention-seeking behavior (Hetherington, 1979).

The differential effects at various ages are more difficult to conceptualize. Kalter and Rembar (1981), in seeking to understand the significance of the child's age on the effects of divorce, have proposed three viewpoints often found in the literature. First, the cumulative effects hypothesis holds that the earlier the divorce occurs in the life of the child, the greater the psychological impact will be. Second, the critical stage hypothesis suggests that at certain times the child's development may be more vulnerable to the particular problems caused by divorce. For example, during the Oedipal phase, the absence of an appropriate figure for same sex identification may have greater significance. Third, there is the recency hypothesis which holds that most reactions are likely to occur immediately following the divorce, with little or no long-term effects.

It is apparent that age has to be seen in relation to another question, that is, Are there both short-term and long-term effects? For example, Kalter and Rembar (1981) found that age at the time of divorce was unrelated to overall level of adjustment. However, the child's age was found to be associated with different types of specific emotional reactions. They found that when divorce occurred before the age of two and a half years, separation-related difficulties occurred during latency; divorce during the Oedipal phase showed the greatest effect in an adolescent group.

The short-term effects at different age levels were also found to vary considerably. Wallerstein and Kelly (1974, 1975, 1976), in a series of studies of more than 100 children from divorced families, found the following characteristic responses at various ages: (a) young preschoolers (two and a half to three and a quarter years) exhibited regressive behaviors; (b) middle preschoolers (three and three quarters to four and three quarters years) displayed irritability, aggressive behavior, self-blame, and bewilderment; (c) older preschoolers (five to six years) showed increased anxiety and aggressive behavior; (d) younger latency-aged children (seven to eight years) responded with sadness, grieving, fear, fantasies of responsibility and reconciliation, anger, and loyalty to both parents; (e) older latency-aged children (nine to ten years) showed feelings of loss, rejection, helplessness, loneliness, shame, anger, and loyalty conflicts; and (f) adolescents (11 years and older) showed sadness, shame, embarrassment, anxiety about the future and marriage, worry, individuation from parents, and withdrawal.

Hetherington (1979) believes that most children can cope with and adapt to the short-term crisis of divorce within a few years; however, if the stress situation is prolonged, developmental disruptions may occur. Moreover, she sees important developmental differences between young children and adolescents. The young child has a tendency to blame himself in interpreting the divorce. He is also more likely to hold distorted perceptions of the parent's behavior, and to equate the separation with total abandonment (Tessman, 1978; Wallerstein and Kelly, 1974, 1975). While most adolescents will experience initial pain and anger when their parents divorce, when the immediate crisis is over they are more able to assign responsibility for the divorce, and to cope with other practical exigencies (Wallerstein and Kelly, 1974, 1975).

In a major nationwide study designed to assess the impact of parental divorce, Guidubaldi, Cleminshaw, Perry, and McLoughlin (1983), reported on over 300 children from divorced families in first, third, and fifth grades in school, and a number of randomly selected controls from intact families. When examining differences between children from divorced and intact families, these investigators found that important differences emerged in both social-emotional and academic-intellectual criteria. Intact family children showed better classroom behavior, were absent less frequently, showed higher peer popularity, demonstrated more internal locus of control, and had higher full scale IQ, reading, and spelling achievement scores. They also found that divorced-family children were far more likely to have been previously referred to a school psychologist, to be in programs for reading difficulties, and to have repeated a grade in school.

By examining the differences within the divorced-family group, the authors were able to comment on the influence of sex and age as mediators. One of the most powerfully demonstrated findings was that in divorced-family households, girls were consistently better adjusted than boys. They were also less likely to have repeated a grade in school. Somewhat surprisingly, the authors found that first graders showed far fewer adverse effects than fifth graders. In general, the younger children seemed to show better adjustment than the older children.

Finally, the investigators found that characteristics of both the home and school environments could help to ameliorate the detrimental effects of divorce.

In conclusion, it is worth remembering that while divorce is always a painful experience, there are times when it is the best solution to a destructive family relationship, and it is by no means inevitable that children will show extreme responses. There is a wide range of variability in its effects on children. Hetherington (1979) addresses that issue succinctly:

> . . . investigators are beginning to examine the interplay among situational factors, stresses, and support systems. However, even when these factors are comparable, wide variability in the quality and intensity of responses and the adaptation of children to divorce remains. Some children exhibit severe or sustained disruptions in development, others seem to sail through a turbulent divorce and stressful aftermath

> and emerge as competent, well-functioning individuals (p. 852).

Hospitalization of the Child

Like the other major stressful life events which we have discussed, the age of the child at the time of the hospital admission may be one of the most important factors to consider in predicting the severity of the stress effects. Rutter (1981) maintains that while hospital admissions rarely provoke emotional disturbance in older children, numerous studies in the literature show that many, but not all, preschool children show emotional adjustment problems in reaction to the event. Distress is most marked between six months and four years of age (Schaffer and Callender, 1959). In addition, the length of hospitalization seems to be important. When young children experience hospitalization of a week or longer, they are likely to show some emotional adjustment reaction (Douglas, 1975). While such disturbance may persist for some time after the discharge, Rutter (1981) concludes that the effects are usually short-term, and that longer lasting effects are unusual.

In discussing the possible long-term effects, Rutter observes that one admission during the preschool years has no association with later emotional disorder, but multiple admissions are associated with increased risk for later disorder (Quinton and Rutter, 1976). He theorizes that the first admission, while it does not lead to disorder, may predispose the child to react adversely the second time he is hospitalized.

Younger children seem especially vulnerable to the effects of hospitalization for a number of reasons. Hospitalization during these years is liable to be disruptive to the developing attachment bonds being formed between the child and his parents. Younger children are more likely to hold distorted perceptions interpreting the hospitalization as rejection and abandonment by the parents. They are more likely to harbor irrational fears, particularly concerning the medical equipment and procedures. The unfamiliar and frightening environment, and parental anxiety, may also contribute to more pronounced effects. Rutter (1981) points out that any efforts to reduce the latter two factors will significantly alleviate the effects of stress on the child.

SUMMARY

The effects of stress on children may be physical, psychological, and/or behavioral. General physiological changes are brought about by the body's stress reaction. In the case of prolonged or severe stress, these changes can affect the health of the child. In some cases specific physical reactions form clusters of symptoms that seem to be associated with stress. Once these psychosomatic disorders are established, the symptoms seem to be exacerbated or mitigated by emotional changes.

The psychological and behavioral effects of stress in children have been demonstrated in a number of studies, particularly those of extreme conditions, as found in the literature on disasters. Specific stressful life events of children offer other opportunities to observe the effects of stress, and to gain some understanding of these factors that serve to influence those effects. Chapter 4 is concerned with the study of those mediating factors in the stress experience.

REFERENCES

Achenbach, T. M., and Lewis, M. A proposed model for clinical research and its application to encopresis and enuresis. J Am Acad Child Psychiatry, 1971, 10, 535-554.

Alexander, F. Psychosomatic medicine. New York: Norton, 1950.

Arthur, B., and Kemme, M. L. Bereavement in childhood. J Child Psychol Psychiatry, 1964, 5, 37-49.

Bakwin, H. Enuresis in children. J Pediatr, 1961, 58, 806-819.

Beitchman, J., and Dielman, T. Predicting hospitalization in child psychiatry: The influence of diagnosis and demographic variables. J Clin Child Psychol, 1982, Sum Vol 11 (2), 116-117.

Bendikson, R., and Fulton, R. Death and the child: An anterospective test of the childhood bereavement and later behavior disorder hypothesis. Omega, 1975, 6 (1), 45-49.

Bernstein, L., and Purcell, K. Institutional treatment of asthmatic children. In W. H. Scheer (Ed.), The asthmatic child: Psychosomatic approaches to problems and treatment. New York: Harper & Row, 1963.

Birtchnell, J. Early parent death in relation to size and constitution of sibling. Acta Psychiatr Scand, 1971, 47, 250-270.

Black, D. What happens to bereaved children? Ther Ed, 1974, 2, 15-20.

Black, D. The bereaved child. J Child Psychol Psychiatry, 1978, 19, 287-292.

Blaufarb, H., and Levine, J. Crisis intervention in an earthquake. Social Work, July, 1972, 16-19.

Block, J. Further considerations of psychosomatic predisposing factors in allergy. Psychosom Med, 1968, 30, 202-208.

Block, J., Jennings, P., Harvey, E., and Simpson, E. Interaction between allergic potential and psychopathology in childhood. Psychosom Med, 1964, 26, 307-320.

Bruch, H. Eating disorders: Obesity, anorexia nervosa and the person within. New York: Basic Books, 1973.

Bruch, H. The golden cage: The enigma of anorexia nervosa. Cambridge, Mass.: Harvard University Press, 1978.

Caplan, M. G., and Douglas, V. I. Incidence of parental loss in children with depressed mood. J Child Psychol Psychiatry, 1969, 10, 225-244.

Crisp, A. H. Anorexia nervosa: Let me be. New York: Grune and Stratton, 1980.

Davidson, M., and Silverberg, M. Ulcerative colitis. In A. M. Rudolph (Ed.), Pediatrics, 17th ed. East Norwalk, Conn.: Appleton-Century-Crofts, 1982.

Douglas, J. Early hospitalization admission and later disturbances of behavior and learning. Dev Med Child Neurol, 1975, 17, 456-480.

Duncan, D. Stress and children: A theoretical overview. Paper presented at the annual meeting of the American Alliance for Health, Physical Education, Recreation and Dance, Minneapolis, 1983.

Ehrensing, R., and Weitzman, E. The mother-daughter relationship in anorexia nervosa. Psychosom Med, 1970, 32 (2), 201-208.

Epstein, G., Weitz, W., Roback, H., and McKee, E. Research on bereavement: A selective and critical review. Compr Psychiatry, 1975, 16 (6), 537-546.

Felner, R. D., Ginter, M. A., Boike, M. F., and Cowen, E. L. Parental death or divorce and the school adjustment of young children. Am J Community Psychol, 1981, 9, 181-190.

Felner, R. D., Stolberg, A., and Cowen, E. L. Crises events and school mental health referral patterns of young children. J Consult Clin Psychol, 1975, 43, 305-310.

Finch, S. M., and Hansen, R. C. Treatment of psychophysiological disorders. In G. P. Sholevar et al. (Eds.), Emotional disorders in children and adolescents. New York: Spectrum Books, 1980.

Garfinkle, P. E., and Garner, D. M. Anorexia nervosa: A multidimensional perspective. New York: Brunner/Mazel, 1982.

Gesten, E. L., Scher, K., and Cowen, E. L. Judged school problems and competencies of referred children with varying family background characteristics. J Abnorm Child Psychol, 1978, 6 (2), 247-255.

Goetz, P. Anorexia nervosa: A follow-up study. Am J Orthopsychiatry, 1977, 47 (4), 597-603.

Gottschalk, L. Vulnerability to "stress." Am J Psychother, 1983, 37 (1), 5-23.

Graham, R., Rutter, M., Yule, W., and Pless, I. Childhood asthma: A psychosomatic disorder? Some epidemiological considerations. Br J Prev Soc Med, 1967, 21, 78-85.

Grossberg, S. H., and Crandall, L. Father loss and father absence in preschool children. Clin Social Work J, 1978, 6, 123-134.

Guidubaldi, J., Climinshaw, H. K., Perry, J. D., and McLoughlin, C. S. The impact of parental divorce on children: Report of the nationwide NASP study. School Psychol Rev, 1983, 7 (3), 300-323.

Hamilton, C. Eating disorders in adolescence. Ment Health Soc, 1975, 2, 243-247.

Hetherington, E. M. Effects of father absence on personality development in adolescent daughters. Dev Psychol, 1972, 72, 313-326.

Hetherington, E. M. Divorce: A child's perspective. Am Psychol, 1979, 34, 851-858.

Jacobs, M. A., Anderson, L. S., Elsman, H. D., Muller, J., and Friedman, S. Interaction of psychologic and biologic predisposing factors in allergic disorders. Psychosom Med, 1967, 2, 572-585.

Kalter, N., and Rembar, J. The significance of a child's age at the time of parental divorce. Am J Orthopsychiatry, 1981, 51, 85-100.

Kirkpatrick, J., Samuels, S., Jones, H., and Zweibelson, J. Bereavement and school adjustment. J School Psychol, 1965, 3 (4), 58-63.

Lapouse, R., and Monk, M. A. Fears and worries in a representative sample of children. Am J Orthopsychiatry, 1959, 29, 803-813.

Lifshitz, M. Long range effects of father's loss: The cognitive complexity of bereaved children and their school adjustment. Br J Med Psychol, 1976, 49, 189-197.

Lovibond, S., and Coote, M. Enuresis. In C. Costello (Ed.), Symptoms of psychopathology. New York: Wiley, 1969.

Lyketsos, G., Arapakis, G., Psaras, M., Photiou, I., and Blackburn, I. Psychological characteristics of hypertensive and ulcer patients. J Psychosom Res, 1982, 26, 255-262.

Mahoney, D. Studies of enuresis: Incidence of obstructive lesions and pathophysiology of enuresis. J Urol, 1971, 106, 951-955.

Markusen, E., and Fulton, R. Childhood bereavement and behavior disorders: A critical review. Omega, 1971, 2, 107-117.

Minuchin, S., Rosman, B., and Baker, L. Psychosomatic families. Cambridge, Mass.: Harvard University Press, 1978.

Mullins, L. L., Siegel, L. J., and Hodges, K. K. Cognitive and life event correlates of depressive symptoms in children. Paper presented at the Annual Meeting of the American Psychological Association, Washington, 1982.

Newman, J. Children of disaster: Clinical observations at Buffalo Creek. Am J Psychiatry, 1976, 133, 306-312.

Oppel, W., Harper, P., and Rowland, V. The age of attaining bladder control. J Pediatr, 1968, 42, 614-626.

Pattison, E. M. The fatal myth of death in the family. Am J Psychiatry, 1976, 133, 674-678.

Purcell, K. Childhood asthma: The role of family relationships, personality and emotions. In A. Davids (Ed.), Child personality and psychopathology: Current topics. Vol. 2. New York: Wiley, 1975.

Purcell, K., Brady, K., Chai, H., Muser, J., Molk, L., Gordon, N., and Means, J. The effect on asthma in children of experimental separation from the family. Psychosom Med, 1969, 31, 144-164.

Quinton, D., and Rutter, M. Early hospital admissions and later disturbances of behavior: An attempted replication of Douglas' findings. Dev Med Child Neurol, 1976, 18, 447-459.

Rappaport, D., Howard, G., and Flint, S. Is there a relationship between allergy and learning disabilities? J School Health, 1976, 46, 139-141.

Rees, L. The importance of psychological, allergic, and infective factors in childhood asthma. J Psychosom Res, 1963, 17, 181-190.

Rees, L. The significance of parental attitudes in childhood asthma. J Psychosom Res, 1963, 7, 181-190.

Rose, R. M., Hurst, M. W., and Herd, J. A. Cardiovascular and endocrine responses to work and the risk for psychiatric symptomatology among air traffic controllers. In J. E. Barrett (Ed.), Stress and mental disorder. New York: Raven Press, 1979.

Rutter, M. Children of sick parents. Oxford: Oxford University Press, 1966.

Rutter, M. Stress, coping and development: Some issues and some questions. J Child Psychol Psychiatry, 1981, 22, 323-356.

Rutter, M., Yule, W., and Graham, P. Enuresis and behavioral deviance: Some epidemiological considerations. In I. Kolvin, R. MacKeith, and S. Meadow (Eds.), Bladder control in enuresis. London: William Heinemann, 1973.

Sandler, I. N., and Block, M. Life stress and maladaptation of children. Am J Community Psychol, 1979, 7, 425-440.

Sandberg, B., and Bliding, A. Duodenal ulcers in army trainees during basic military training. J Psychosom Res, 1975, 20, 61-74.

Schaffer, H. R., and Callender, W. M. Psychological effects of hospitalization in infancy. Pediatrics, 1959, 24, 528-539.

Selvini-Palazzoli, M. Self-starvation: From individual to family therapy in treating anorexia nervosa. New York: Jason Aronson, 1978.

Selye, H. Stress in health and disease. Woburn, Mass.: Butterworth, 1976.

Shepherd, D. M., and Barraclough, B. M. The aftermath of parental suicide for children. Br J Psychiatry, 1976, 129, 267-276.

Shinn, M. Father absence and children's cognitive development. Psychol Bull, 1978, 85, 295-324.

Siegel, D. J. Separation-loss events, self concept, locus of control, and children's effective functioning in school. Unpublished doctoral dissertation, University of Pittsburth, 1981.

Silber, E., Perry, S. E., and Bloch, D. A. Patterns of parent-child interaction in a disaster. Am J Psychiatry, 1957, 21, 159-167.

Silverman, S. M., and Silverman, P. R. Parent-child communication in widowed families. Am J Psychother, 1979, 33, 428-441.

Sperling, M. Asthma in children: An evaluation of concepts and therapies. J Am Acad Child Psychiatry, 1968, 7, 44-58.

Stein, Z., and Susser, M. Nocturnal enuresis as a phenomenon of institutions. Dev Med Child Neurol, 1966, 8, 677-685.

Stein, Z., and Susser M. Social factors in the development of sphincter control. Dev Med Child Neurol, 1967, 9, 692-706.

Tessman, L. H. Children of parting parents. New York: Aronson, 1978.

Trombini, G., Baccarani, C., Rossi, N., and Umilta, C. Experimental stress and cystomanometric recordings of patients with primary enuresis: A preliminary report. Percep Mot Skills, 1982, 54, 771-777.

Wallerstein, J. S., and Kelly, J. B. The effects of parental divorce: The adolescent experience. In E. Anthony and C. Koupernik (Eds.), The child and his family (Vol. 3). New York: Wiley, 1974.

Wallerstein, J. S., and Kelly, J. B. The effects of parental divorce: Experiences of the preschool child. J Am Acad Child Psychiatry, 1975, 14, 600-616.

Wallerstein, J. S., and Kelly, J. B. The effects of parental divorce: Experiences of the child in later latency. Am J Orthopsychiatry, 1976, 46, 256-269.

Werry, J. S. Psychosomatic disorders, psychogenic symptoms and hospitalization. In H. C. Quay and J. S. Werry (Eds.), Psychopathological disorders of childhood (2nd Ed.). New York: Wiley, 1979.

Wolff, C. T., Friedman, S. B., Hofer, M. A., and Mason, J. W. Relationships between psychological defense and mean urinary 17-hydroxycorticosteroid excretion rates: A predictive study of parents of children with leukemia. Psychosom Med, 1964, 26, 576-591.

4

MEDIATORS OF STRESS

While earlier studies tended to examine the relationship between stress as a noxious stimulus and some disease or discomfort as a response, the limitations of this simplistic two-variable design became increasingly apparent (Coyne and Lazarus, 1980; Jenkins, 1979). It was obvious that there were individual differences that might account for the fact that two individuals, exposed to identical stressful stimuli, might respond in widely divergent manners. This led to the investigation of individual differences in stress research. Dohrenwend and Dohrenwend (1974) put it this way:

> A major question, and for some investigators the central problem concerning the effects of stressful life events, grows out of the observation that one individual may become ill and another remain healthy after both experience the same life event. The most general formulation of the research question generated by these individual differences is: What are the factors that mediate the impact of stressful life events on the individual? (p. 316).

This chapter will be concerned with examining the research designed to investigate the mediators of stress, that is, those factors that serve as moderator variables by increasing or lessening the impact of stress.

A REVIEW OF THE RESEARCH

A number of writers have attempted to identify and classify the moderators of stress. Jenkins (1979) examined the different capabilities of individuals to adapt to specific kinds of stressors. He relates their psychosocial adaptive capacities to the "host resistance" concept of medicine. He sees ego strength, problem-solving ability, flexibility, and social skills as the psychological counterparts to host resistance. Antonovsky (1974), in a similar way, views the mediating set of variables between life crises and health as "resistance resources." Dohrenwend and Dohrenwend (1974), in discussing individual differences in response to stress, classify the mediating processes into physiological, psychological, and social.

Rutter (1981) points out that the personal qualities and characteristics that an individual brings to the stress interaction are likely to be important. He lists such variables as age, sex, genetic factors, temperament, intelligence, and problem-solving skills as being relevant. He also discusses the importance of social group identity, cognitive appraisal, and other factors that have been found to mitigate the effects of stress.

Christensen (1981), in discussing moderator variables, points to the key role of individual perception as important in determining the impact of stress. Particularly, the amount of perceived control over events seems important. Stimuli are seen as more aversive if they are perceived as outside of the person's control. He also lists personality characteristics (that is, the hard-driving, competitively hostile, type A personality), demographic variables (for example, age, sex, race, and socioeconomic class), and social supports as relevant moderator variables.

Zautra and Beier (1978) investigated the role of social conditions and perceived quality of life on the part of the individual in helping to lessen the debilitating effects of stress by facilitating adjustment. Since adverse social conditions such as low income and lack of education were thought to reduce a person's capacity for adaptation, the authors hypothesized that favorable social conditions and life qualities would influence psychological well-being, and be especially valuable to those experiencing crises in their lives. They found that life crises were associated with psychological adjustment, with social conditions (income, age, marital status, education, and religious participation), and quality of life (family, personal, income, and overall) having significant effects.

Rabkin and Struening (1976), in their review of the research literature on life events, stress, and illness, classified mediators into two broad groups: individual characteristics and external variables. Their review found considerable support for the common observation that one of the most critical factors in determining the impact of stress is the individual's perception. Perception, in turn, depends on personal characteristics that are called upon to aid in appraising the threat associated with the event or situation. Factors such as biological and psychological threshold sensitivities, intelligence, verbal skills, morale, personality type, psychological defenses, past experience, and a sense of mastery over one's fate are relevant. Demographic characteristics such as age, education, income, and occupation may also contribute.

Rabkin and Struening go on to summarize the individual characteristics this way:

> The effects of most personal variables in mediating stressful conditions are fairly obvious: persons with more skills, assets, and resources, and with more versatile defenses and broader experience tend to fare better. In general, the more competence individuals have demonstrated in the past, the more likely it is that they will cope adaptively with a current stressor (p. 1018).

For Rabkin and Struening the external variables are those buffers and supports found in the social environment. Individual and group social identity and status, the degree of role conflict, the availability of social supports or networks, the degree of social isolation, and status inconsistency have all been identified as external variables that mediate the effect of exposure to stressful events.

While a number of writers have discussed the general role of the mediators of stress, there have been relatively few studies that dealt with those factors which might be most relevant for children.

Egeland et al. (1980) used a discriminate function analysis to investigate the possible effect of life stress on mothers. They were interested in finding out if mothers with high life stress were more likely to abuse their children. They found that only a minority of their stressed mothers mistreated their children, and that they differed from the majority of mothers with similar high stress scores who did not abuse their children on a number of factors. Those who mistreated their children were found to have certain personality characteristics, poorer patterns of interaction with their infants, and less understanding of the demands of parenthood.

Silber et al. (1957) interviewed parents and their children in the aftermath of a tornado. They were particularly interested in the pattern of parent-child interaction. They pointed out that the child, especially in a disaster situation, relies on the parent for support. They reasoned that what the parent provided at such times was a ready-built perception or structure of the event for the child. Blaufarb and Levine (1972) have also pointed to the importance of parental support during times of crisis.

Moore (1975), in reviewing work conducted at the University of London, described moderators as those having to do with parental characteristics as well as constitutional factors of the child. Characteristics of the parents were: (1) the personality, self-satisfaction, and adjustment of the parents; (2) their relation to each other; (3) their feelings toward the child (warm positive feelings were seen as best); and (4) their own reactions to stress. Among the constitutional factors, Moore included genetic, temperamental, and perinatal factors, such as anoxia, which he maintains tends to make the child more sensitive to noxious stimuli.

Gersten et al. (1977), in investigating the nature of the relationship between stressful life events and psychological disorder in children, found that events, in and of themselves, did not significantly contribute to behavioral pathology. Rather an alternative hypothesis, that sociocultural factors confound the relationship, seemed to be supported.

A summary of the findings of these and other studies is presented in Table 4.1, which lists the major factors identified as mediators of childhood stress. A more detailed examination of each factor might be helpful.

TABLE 4.1

Mediators of Childhood Stress

Mediating Factors	Relevant Citations
Individual characteristics	
Perception of threat; appraisal	Christensen (1981); Coyne and Lazarus (1980); Endler (1975); Magnusson (1982); Rabkin and Struening (1976); Rutter (1981)
Psychological adjustment and self-esteem	Jenkins (1979); Pearlin and Schooler (1978); Rabkin and Struening (1976); Wills and Langner (1980); Zautra and Beier (1978)
Age	Christensen (1981); Magnusson (1982); Rabkin and Struening (1976); Rutter (1981); Zautra and Beier (1978)
Perceived control; sense of mastery; competency	Christensen (1981); Mandler (1982); Moos and Billings (1982); Rabkin and Struening (1976); Sarason and Sarason (1981); Wills and Langner (1980)
Problem-solving abilities and previous experience	Jenkins (1979); Kendall and Hollon (1980); Rabkin and Struening (1976); Rutter (1981); Wills and Langner (1980)
Parental characteristics	
Psychological adjustment	Egeland et al. (1980); Moore (1975)
Good marital relations	Moore (1975)
Realistic, supportive attitude toward child	Blaufarb and Levine (1972); Moore (1969); Silber et al. (1957)
Social factors	
Social support network	Christensen (1981); Cobb (1976); Rabkin and Struening (1976); Sarason and Sarason (1981)
Social group identity	Rabkin and Struening (1976); Rutter (1981); Wills and Langner (1980)

Perception of Threat; Appraisal

Antonovsky (1974) has remarked on the generally held view that a key role is played by the individual's perception of the potentially stressful event: ". . . if anything has been learned in the study of stressful life events, it is that what is important for the consequences is the subjective perception of the meaning of the event rather than its objective character" (p. 246).

One of the most detailed analyses of the perceptual process has been made by Lazarus and his associates (Coyne and Lazarus, 1980). Lazarus sees the process as a cognitive-phenomenological one which he calls cognitive appraisal. Appraisal refers to the evaluative process that imbues a situational encounter with meaning (Holyrod and Lazarus, 1982). Lazarus emphasizes the dynamic, transactional nature of this process. It is the individual's cognitive appraisal of the threat that fuses certain personal and situational variables, along with the environmental responses, which then feed back for subsequent analysis.

For Lazarus, cognitive appraisal involves continually reevaluated judgments regarding the demand and the resources available to the person in meeting that demand. The process is in two phases. Primary appraisal answers the question, "Am I okay or in trouble?" At this phase, the appraisal may involve harm-loss, threat, or challenge. For Lazarus the distinction between threat and harm-loss is that the former implies a future event, while the latter refers to damage already done. Secondary appraisal can be seen as the answer to the question, "What can I do about it?" This phase involves judgments concerning coping resources, options, and constraints. The distinction between these two phases is not always clear, and they may even fuse.

Endler (1980) has also focused on the perception of the situation as the prime determinant of the individual's response. In his interactionist approach, he advocates the investigation of how perceptual factors in situations affect reactions.

Magnusson (1982), citing the work of Lazarus, Endler, and others, sees the need to distinguish between the actual and the perceived environments. He points out that the actual environment has been historically a major concern of behavioral psychology, and is today the subject of study of environmental psychology. Early stress research also employed the actual environment approach.

However, there has been another consistent strain in the history of psychology that called attention to the meaning of the environment, that is, how it is perceived, interpreted, and cognitively represented in the minds of individuals (see Magnusson, 1982, for a review). This approach is particularly relevant to interactional psychology, and therefore to stress research based on interactionist models.

Both approaches are necessary in studying stress:

> For effective theories and models for behavior in relation to the environment in general (and in relation to stressful situations), we obviously need both the actual and the perceived environment approach. . . . Two of the most important issues in psychology are the way an individual's conceptions of the external world are formed on the basis of information about the environment "as it is" and the way these conceptions function in relation to the actual, objective conditions at a specific time and place (p. 233).

In stress research these two approaches define the types of situations. Actual situations pertain to that part of the environment that is accessible in a relatively stable fashion to sensory perception. The perceived situation is the situation as it is perceived, interpreted, and represented cognitively.

Psychological Adjustment and Self-Esteem

While many writers seem to agree that the overall mental health of the individual influences the effects of stress, that variable is usually not well defined. Jenkins (1979) speaks of "ego strength," and Zautra and Beier (1978) of a "personal quality" reflecting, among other things, self-satisfaction.

Rabkin and Struening (1976), in their review, cite a number of psychological variables including "morale" and "personality type," as mediating factors. While several authors suggest that personality type is important, few specify the actual traits that might be relevant. The one major exception on which there is some agreement seems to involve the type A personality (Friedman and Rosenman, 1959). This is the ambitious, aggressive, hard-driving, competitively hostile personality which has been found to be of high risk for coronary heart disease (Christensen, 1981; Friedman and Rosenman, 1974; Sparacino, 1979).

Minter and Kimball (1980) cite the work of Jacobs and associates (1966, 1967) to show that the dependent personality type is susceptible to disease. Their dependent personality was defined by measures on maternal domination, parental rejection, exaggerated dependency, and neurotic emotional lability. Those subjects with many of those factors present were found to have more allergic reactions than a control group.

Wills and Langner (1980) argue that stress must be considered in terms of the social and psychological processes that produce it. For them, low self-esteem and incompetence are directly linked to a lack of emotional support. They maintain that when people are exposed to stress, those with social supports of various kinds have much lower levels of symptomatology when compared to those lacking social supports (compare Cobb, 1976; Rabkin and Struening, 1976). They go on to suggest that part of the reason for the marked effect of social support is that supporting persons offer reassurance and acceptance of the stressed person, confirming that he is "esteemed and valued." An increased sense of esteem, in turn, increases the resistance to the effects of stress.

Age

A number of studies have included age as a demographic variable in assessing the impact of stress (Rabkin and Struening, 1976; Zautra and Beier, 1978). Ilfeld (1980) reported a positive correlation between age and psychosomatic disorders; while Christensen (1981) reported a negative correlation. Magnusson (1982) has found that children and adolescents at various ages perceive the nature of a threat differently. He found that a shift occurs from preadolescence to postadolescence from an awareness of threat based on the manifest characteristics of the situation, to one based on the latent characteristics.

While there seems to be some general agreement that children, because of their immaturity, are more vulnerable to stressful events and situations than are adults, the influence of age on the impact of stress is unclear. There is a considerable body of literature in human development and in psychodynamic psychology that suggests that there are certain times during development when the individual may show particular readiness for certain experiences (for example, language acquisition), and be particularly vulnerable to specific disrupters. For example, Bowlby (1969) has shown that human attachment bonds typically develop in the age range from six months to six years. He maintains that loss of the mother figure during this critical time increases the chances for pathological personality development.

Psychodynamic theorists have also pointed to the early childhood years as a time of particular vulnerability to trauma which may lay the groundwork for adult mental disorders.

Rutter (1981), discussing the importance of age in children's stress responses, illustrates the effect by the example of hospitalization. He maintains that children between six months and four years of age are likely to show the most distress when hospitalized. He relates this distress to the developmentally important task of forming selective attachments. He concludes that it is the interference with attachment implicit in hospitalization that constitutes one of the features making it so stressful.

In a similar way bereavement, another specific stress situation, has been found to have different effects on children, depending in part on their age. Rutter reports findings that suggest that immediate grief reactions are both milder and of shorter duration in young children, as opposed to adolescents or adults (Bowlby, 1980; Kliman, 1968; Rutter, 1966). Rutter goes on to comment on the differential effects of stress, based on the age of occurrence, by maintaining that the meaning and impact of events may be influenced by whether or not they occurred in what are commonly seen as "appropriate" times in the life cycle. He concludes that age is an important variable for some types of stress events, but even in those for which it is important, the effects vary according to the variety of the event.

Perceived Control; Sense of Mastery; Competence

Christensen (1981) has called the perception of personal control over life events a powerful variable influencing the stressfulness of those events. It has been shown that when aversive stimuli seem to be outside of the individual's control, they become even more stressful (Lefcourt, 1973). Conversely, the perception of personal control over events has been found to reduce the amount of anxiety associated with them (Seligman, 1975).

Mandler (1982) hypothesizes that a sense of mastery is important because it colors the cognitive interpretation of our world. Since it is generally seen as good to be in control of our world, the world is appraised as good, and the emotional tone will be more positive. In this context, the actual control of environmental events may be largely irrelevant, as it is the subjective sense of control that is important. Such a sense of mastery reduces the deleterious effects of stress and alleviates the subjective sense of emotional disturbance.

Wills and Langner (1980) relate the perceived lack of control to an element of unpredictability, which makes events particularly stressful. They point out that when people are placed in situations where aversive events occur unpredictably and outside of their personal control, the result is feelings of helplessness, incompetence, frustration, depression, anxiety, and fatigue (Miller and Norman, 1979). Myers, Lindenthal, and Pepper (1971) found that negative events outside of the control of the individual were particularly important for discriminating subjects with high versus low scores on psychiatric impairment.

Rotter (1966, 1975) did much to promote interest in the construct of locus of control. For Rotter, locus of control reflects the belief that reinforcement follows contingent on one's own behavior. A situation of external control is perceived when reinforcement is seen as following some action of the individual, although it is not contingent on that action. In such cases the individual may attribute reinforcement to chance, luck, fate, or the control of powerful others in his environment. Locus of control is placed on a continuum with each individual having some degree of internality/externality in his perceptions.

Locús of control beliefs have been found to be mediators of adaptive functioning in children. For example, internal children when compared to external children have been found to show greater academic achievement, higher self-esteem, less anxiety, less emotional maladjustment, greater persistence, and greater ability to evaluate and use new information (Gordon et al., 1981; Joe, 1971; Phares, 1976; Nowicki and Strickland, 1973).

Closely related to the sense of mastery is the construct of competence. Competence is a rather broad concept related to mastery. White (1963) has defined competence as the individual's existing capacity to effectively interact with the environment. It depends on an accumulation of interactions with the environment and so is related to previous experience. White sees signal anxiety as arising when threat exceeds one's sense of competence, that is, the individual's perception that he can do something about the situation.

In general, the more competence individuals have demonstrated in the past, the more likely it is that they will cope adequately with a current stressor (Rabkin and Struening, 1976).

A number of writers have specifically identified competence as being an important mediator for children in stress situations (compare Garmezy, 1973), and their work will be reviewed later in this chapter.

Problem-Solving Abilities and Previous Experience

The ability to solve problems is a complex one which depends on general intelligence, the ability to think abstractly, reasoning skills, generalization and discrimination abilities, memory, and past experiences. Spivak, Platt, and Shure (1976) have identified three main elements of problem solving: recognizing the existence of a problem, generating possible solutions, and evaluating the alternatives and selecting the optimal solution.

Rabkin and Struening (1976) maintain that individuals with more skills, assets, and resources, along with broader experience, tend to be able to cope more effectively. They go on to argue that the more experience these individuals may have had with a specific stressor, the more likely their present coping responses will be effective.

In a similar way, Rutter (1981) sees intelligence and problem-solving skills among the potentially relevant characteristics that the individual brings to the stress situation. He suggests that children with higher intelligence may be more resistant to stress, and he speculates that this may, in turn, be related to their greater problem-solving skills.

The Role of the Parents

Because of the generally recognized crucial role that parents play in interpreting life events for children, providing models and giving them emotional support, their individual personalities, as well as their relations to each other and to their children, they are important as mediators. Moore (1975) calls parental adjustment a key factor in the production of well-adjusted children. He cites evidence of problems of children resulting from situations in which a parent was diagnosed as mentally ill. Studies have also found a relationship between parental, particularly maternal, mood (such as depression and hostility) and adjustment problems in children (Shearman, 1968). Other studies have shown that maternal satisfaction is important to the child's development (Yarrow, 1962).

In comparing stressed mothers who had mistreated their children with a similar group who had not, Egeland et al. (1980) found personality differences. Stressed mothers who mistreated their children were found to have higher scores on aggression and anxiety, and lower scores on succorance.

Some idea of the role of parents as mediators in stress situations can be seen by the analysis of traumatic events. For example, the considerable contribution that parents can make was illustrated by Silber et al. (1957) in their analysis of parent-child interaction when a tornado struck the town of Vicksburg, Mississippi. Their analysis included the reaction of the parent with the child at the time of impact, communication between parent and child about the disaster, and the parent's response to the child's behavior in the aftermath of the disaster. They concluded that one essential role involves influencing the child's integration of the experience. Parents help their children to order, structure, understand, and integrate the experience into the child's own frame of reference, so that it does not remain an awful, mysterious, threatening memory. Verbalization facilitates the process by providing meaning to an experience, even as it provides a channel for affective discharge.

In addition, supportive parents were those who were aware of their child's need to temporarily regress during the stressful situation. They were accepting of the child's behavior, allowing some regression, although they controlled the timing, seeking to return the child to previous levels of behavior as soon as reasonable. They attended to their own needs and anticipated their child's needs by providing active support.

While no one pattern of child handling seemed better in all cases, the authors felt that whatever patern was chosen, it would be more successful if it was characterized by consistency. They concluded that

> Granting the merits of the facilitation of communication, the maintenance of parental roles, and the acceptance of regressive and symptomatic behavior, we felt that, if there was any parental behavior making for a better adjustment in the child, it was probably consistency and lack of confusion (Silber et al., p. 165).

Social Factors

A number of social factors have been suggested as external mediators of stress from the interactionist perspective. In general, the environment provides buffers and social supports to the individual, which affects his experience of stress (Rabkin and Struening, 1976).

Cobb (1976) has reviewed studies indicating that social supports protect individuals in crises from various pathological outcomes. Social supports provide a sense that the individual is accepted, cared for, esteemed, and valued, and that he is a member of a network of mutual obligations.

As has been pointed out above, Wills and Langner (1980) have discussed the interactive nature of self-esteem and social support. They hypothesize that since supporting persons offer reassurance, confirming that the stressed person is esteemed and valued, they contribute directly to self-esteem. They see this as an example of social-psychological processes that counter the low self-esteem and sense of incompetence so detrimental in stress situations.

The most compelling evidence for the importance of social group identity and support network comes from the studies of social isolation (Rabkin and Struening, 1976). Evidence has been found to suggest that those who live alone without involvement with people or organizations are more likely to have a higher risk of a variety of chronic diseases. The much-commented-on "failure to thrive" of some institutionalized children may also be associated with a lack of meaningful interpersonal relations.

Rutter (1981) discusses one aspect of the social supports available to children--the schools. He cites studies of school influences (Rutter et al., 1979) that show that schools vary markedly in rates of disruptive behavior and absenteeism, and these variations are characteristics of the schools themselves. He goes on to conclude that this suggests that schools can be a force for good (or bad) even with children living under conditions of psychosocial disadvantage. He cautions, however, that one cannot conclude from that that it is the effect of the social group that modifies the children's response to stress, since that remains an unproven hypothesis.

VULNERABILITY TO STRESS

The focus on the mediators of stress was sharpened by researchers examining the variables that determined why some children were more vulnerable to stress than others. This interest grew from early work concerned with identifying the factors that placed children in high-risk for adult schizophrenia. The first step was to identify a group of children who might be especially vulnerable to the disease. For example, genetic studies had shown that children of a schizophrenic parent would constitute such a high-risk group. This group could then be studied longitudinally. Their development could be carefully monitored. Should some of these children subsequently develop adult psychopathology, their data could be examined retrospectively and compared against those of children who did not. By such studies it might be possible to identify the precursor signs that point to later disorder (Mednik and Schulsinger, 1973). In the course of their investigations these researchers demonstrated a methodological approach that could be used to study the development of psychopathology (Garmezy, 1981). Initially, the research on present differentiators and future predictors of children at risk had been concerned with the children of psychotic parents (Anthony, 1974). Gradually, other groups began to be added. Disadvantaged children, those who suffered parental loss, adopted children, and children of divorce were to be included in the studies of vulnerable children. It was assumed that these children, by virtue of their unique constitutional or social history, would be likely to show problems of adjustment and ultimately adult psychopathology.

For the most part it appears as though the direct relationship hypothesized between these childhood problems and adult psychopathology failed to materialize. Anthony (1978) summarized the situation by pointing out that while a few children succumbed, about half suffered to greater or lesser degrees and a few "came through mysteriously unscathed." Garmezy (1981) agreed that long-range forecasting applied to vulnerable children left much to be desired. Indeed, he maintained that "more children, if followed into adulthood, are likely to escape our dire predictions than fall victim to them."

Increasingly, it was that subgroup of vulnerable children who showed no evidence of maladjustment that began to interest workers in that field. Anthony (1974) has described these "invulnerable" children this way:

> One is surprised at the absence of disorder in the presence of appalling living conditions, horrifying experiences, chronic physical ailments, and disruptive development. In the presence of all of this, an individual emerges who is energetic, well balanced, and normally active and reactive (pp. 538-539).

Garmezy (1981), in tracing the history of the study of invulnerable (or, as he prefers to call them, "stress-resistant") children, cites the work of Manfred Bleuler. Bleuler (1974) studied a group of high-risk subjects, the offspring of schizophrenic parents, and reported a high percentage of them became mentally healthy adults. He pointed out that the accomplishments of this group were even more remarkable given the emotional, social, and economic hardships with which they began life.

Garmezy and his associates at the University of Minnesota, who had been conducting extensive studies of high-risk children, now began to shift their focus to discover the constructive, growth-oriented forces that characterized the stress-resistant child. Beginning with careful observations of the lives of high-risk children, they sought to identify individual variations that might contribute to self-sufficiency and greater adaptation.

They began by reviewing the literature on disadvantaged children (Garmezy and Nuechterlein, 1972). In their review they concentrated on the findings that described the strengths of such children. In summing up their review of these positive findings, Garmezy makes this point:

> despite the harshness of life that the families encounter, some parents appear to be able to foster or enhance in their children the confidence, self-control, determination, flexibility, and cognitive and social skills that accompany the development of competence and positive adaptation. These appear to be important precursors to the establishment of stress-resistance in children (p. 221).

For Garmezy, the concept of competence has taken on central importance in the study of children at risk. He has made a significant contribution by defining and identifying the indicators of competence in children.

White (1963) has defined competence as the individual's existing capacity to interact effectively with the environment. In his psychodynamic formulation, competence develops from independent ego energy and effectance. It reflects an accumulation of interactions with the environment regardless of motivation. Exploratory and manipulative activity and play enable the child to construct reality, learn flexible controls, and develop a sense of competence. In this way the child's recognition that he can affect his environment in desired ways becomes an important aspect of ego development.

Siegel (1981) has pointed to the parallels between White's description of competence in ego development and the theoretical formulations of stress theory. He quotes White to show that competence can be seen as an adaptive capacity that mediates the impact of stress:

> The use by the ego of anxiety as a signal depends upon a situation being apprehended as one of potential danger. This danger has to be conceived of in terms that include, as one variable, what the person feels he can do about the situation. Danger is spotted when threat exceeds one's sense of competence (White, 1963, p. 40).

White maintains that it is the development of competence that strengthens the ego for its encounters with future threats.

Garmezy has reviewed a number of studies which have identified aspects of competence. He lists six aspects as indexes of competence in the middle years of childhood (Garmezy, 1973):

1. Effectiveness in work, play, and love; satisfactory educational and occupational progress; peer regard and friendships.

2. Healthy expectations and the belief that "good outcomes" will follow from the imposition of effort and initiative; an orientation to success rather than the anticipation of failure in performing tasks; a realistic level of aspiration unbeclouded by unrealistically high or low goal-setting behavior.

3. Self-esteem, feelings of personal worthiness, a proper evaluative set toward self and a sense of "fate control," that is, the belief that one can control events in one's environment rather than be a passive victim of them (an internal as opposed to external locus of control).

4. Self-discipline, as revealed by the ability to delay gratification and to maintain a future-orientedness.

5. Control and regulation of impulsive drives; the ability to adopt a reflective as opposed to an impulsive style in coping with problem situations.

6. The ability to think abstractly; to approach new situations and to be able to attempt alternate solutions to a problem.

While competence seems to have an important role in determining vulnerability to stress, a number of other aspects of this problem are also being explored. Anthony (1974) has pointed to the very beginnings of life, including prenatal influences, as those which might initially determine vulnerability. He reviewed a number of theoretical and research contributions suggesting that constitutionally determined behavior patterns seen in infancy could provide an indicator of the ability to adapt. For example, babies were found to differ widely in their activity levels, the strength of their startle responses, and their avoidance of unpleasant stimuli.

This is consistent with the findings of Thomas, Chess, and Birch (1968) who conducted the New York Longitudinal Study of "normal" families. They found that a child's temperamental influences in early childhood were predictors of later emotional disturbance. Rutter et al. (1973), using similar measures with a group of children one of whose parents was a psychiatric patient, found that children who were highly irregular in their sleeping and eating patterns, whose behavior lacked malleability in that it was difficult to alter, and who were markedly nonfastidious, were more susceptible to stress. He concluded that temperamental features were associated with individual differences in susceptibility to stressful family circumstances.

Still another aspect of the study of vulnerability to stress comes from the psychoanalytic tradition. Freud's insistence that traumatic events in early childhood could lay the groundwork for later adult neuroses has continued to influence the theoretical and research literature. In their search for childhood antecedents to adult disorders, psychoanalytic workers have sometimes disagreed on the relative importance of certain factors (for example, the Oedipus complex), but most hold that events and situations of childhood produce enduring changes in personality and the ability to cope effectively. Gardner (1973) provides an excellent illustration of a psychoanalytic point of view in his contention that basic deprivation in the parent-child love relationship lies at the root of many later disorders.

In his formulation, Gardner has modified Freud's contention that the unresolved Oedipal situation forms the core of neurotic symptom formation. Rather, Gardner contends, it is not so much sexual union with the opposite-sex parent that the child desires so much as it is love and attention undiluted by rivals. While these feelings may be sexually tinged, Gardner maintains they are not sexual, except in the broadest meaning of the term. For Gardner the child who lacks love and attention, or perceives a lack of love and attention, is deprived and vulnerable to later disorder. It is the failure of the child to come to terms with this basic deprivation, and not his failure to resolve his sexual feelings for his parent, that underlies neuroses. Gardner states it this way:

> In my opinion whatever cultural, social and biological factors may be operative in the etiology of neurotic symptoms, parental, and especially maternal, deprivation is essential to their formation.

Gottschalk (1983) has explored other psychodynamic factors that increase vulnerability to the psychological and physiological effects of stress. He uses the example of the genesis of duodenal ulcers to illustrate the interaction of emotional factors with genetic disposition. Ulcer patients show physiological patterns of hyperreactivity and a tendency to hypersecretion of gastric acid. Psychologically they show strong oral dependency. For such individuals the onset of ulcer symptoms is often precipitated by the stress associated with separation from or loss of an emotionally important person. This type of vulnerability is selective since emotional investment and involvement with the parents tends to affect one child rather than another. Expanding on his views, Gottschalk goes on to relate the onset of disease symptoms to emotional disruptions in the family dynamics, particularly consequent on the loss of a significant other person:

> Loss of such significant relationships, followed by a period of inadequate and morbid grief which is then replaced by the disease state, has been traced in ulcerative colitis, rheumatoid arthritis, leukemia, and even anniversary psychosomatic reactions, as well as a variety of other forms of organic decompensation. The more general findings, however, in the family context, are not specifically the loss of a significant object, but a variety of disruptions which upset the emotional balance in the family system (Gottschalk, 1983, p. 13).

Gottschalk concludes his discussion of the psychodynamic factors at work in families by pointing out that emotional disorganization does not affect all members of the family equally, but according to their degree of involvement. Thus certain children may be more vulnerable depending on their involvement in the family dynamics.

Gottschalk (1983) has identified the following factors in a recent review of studies of vulnerability in humans. (Individual citations have been omitted here to increase readability. Interested readers are referred to the original work for detailed references.)

Genetic and congenital predisposition, for example, pepsinogen secretion and duodenal ulcers, cancer and leukemia prone, affective disorders, schizophrenia, average evoked potential reducers or augmenters.

Psychosocial factors: These include early parent loss without prompt replacement with a parental substitute, narrow kinship and social networks, delayed grief reactions, and major life-change and family-change events that increase susceptibility to cancer, infections, and other diseases.

Several recent studies have tested the propositions concerning vulnerability to stress. Solomon and Bromet (1982) tested the vulnerability model of Brown and Harris (1978) which delineates a woman's unemployment, lack of a confiding relationship with husband or male friend, and having three or more children over the age of 14 years as factors contributing to the development of depression in the presence of a provoking stressor. The researchers interviewed 327 mothers living in the area of Three Mile Island after the nuclear accident. They compared their responses with a control group living in a comparable area. The nuclear accident was seen as a provoking stressor. Their results did not support the model, and they concluded that a broader array of vulnerability factors might be necessary to explain stress-induced depression.

To see if a history of certain stressful life events would increase vulnerability in children, Siegel (1981) examined the school functioning of children with a history of separation-loss events using two aspects of competence (locus of control and self-concept) as mediating variables. Following Garmezy's (1981) suggestion that attention should be paid to healthy adaptive functioning rather than to the indicators of maladjustment, Siegel measured effective school functioning using a Health Resources Inventory. The Piers-Harris Self Concept Scale and the Nowicki-Strickland locus of control scale for children were used to measure mediating factors. Using a multiple regression analysis, Siegel found that a history of separation-loss events significantly contributed to a prediction of school functioning with his group of third grade children. Self-concept and locus of control had an additional impact, seen by the increased amount of variance explained when they were entered into the procedure. In all, approximately 21 percent of the variance in school functioning could be attributed to these three variables. The limited but significant amount of variance attributed to these factors suggests that the performance of children with a history of stressful life events may be moderated by certain aspects of competence, but those factors are not sufficient in themselves to explain the differences in school functioning. These findings lead to a similar conclusion to that proposed by Solomon and Bromet (1982), as described above, that is, that a broader range of variables may need to be identified and employed in experimental studies of the mediating factors.

In another study of children, Mullins et al. (1982) examined the relationship of various cognitive and life event variables to depressive symptoms. The variables studied were locus of control, problem-solving ability, and life stress. Several measures were employed, including the Nowicki-Strickland Locus of Control Scale, the Children's Depression Inventory, the Social Means-Ends Problem Solving Procedure, the Emotional Means-End Problem Solving Procedure, The Optional Thinking Test, the Anagram Test, and Coddington's Life Events Scale for Children. Results indicated that higher levels of depressive symptoms were associated with an external locus of control, increased level of life stress, and lower performance levels on an impersonal problem-solving task. The level of depressive symptom was also found to be inversely related to socioeconomic status as measured by father's occupation.

In summary, the search for moderator variables, given impetus by the study of vulnerable children, is continuing. The need to identify those variables, clearly define and operationalize them for experimental work, and examine their interactive effects in a stress paradigm, provides important objectives for future research.

REFERENCES

Anthony, E. J. A risk-vulnerability intervention model for children of psychotic parents. In E. J. Anthony and C. Koupernik (Eds.), _The child in his family: Children at psychiatric risk_ (Vol. 3). New York: Wiley, 1974.

Anthony, E. J. A new scientific region to explore. In E. J. Anthony and C. Koupernik (Eds.), _The child in his family: Vulnerable children_ (Vol. 4). New York: Wiley, 1978.

Antonovsky, A. Conceptual and methodological problems in the study of resistance resources and stressful life events. In B. S. Dohrenwend and B. P. Dohrenwend (Eds.), Stressful life events: Their nature and effects. New York: Wiley, 1974.

Blaufarb, H., and Levine, J. Crisis intervention in an earthquake. Social Work, July, 1972, 16-19.

Bleuler, M. The offspring of schizophrenics. Schizophr Bull, 1974, No. 8, 93-107.

Bowlby, J. Attachment and loss: I. Attachment. London: Hogarth Press, 1969.

Bowlby, J. Attachment and loss: III. Loss, sadness and depression. New York: Basic Books, 1980.

Brown, G., and Harris, T. The social origins of depression: A study of psychiatric disorder in women. London: Tavistock, 1978.

Christensen, J. F. Assessment of stress: Environmental, intrapersonal, and outcomes issues. In R. McReynolds (Ed.), Advances in psychological assessment (Vol. 5). San Francisco, Calif.: Jossey-Bass, 1981.

Cobb, S. Social support as a moderator of life stress. Psychosom Med, 1976, 38, 300-314.

Coyne, J. C., and Lazarus, R. S. Cognitive style, stress perception, and coping. In I. L. Kutash et al. (Eds.), Handbook on stress and anxiety. San Francisco, Calif.: Jossey-Bass, 1980.

Dohrenwend, B. S., and Dohrenwend, B. P. Overview and prospects for research on stressful life events. In B. S. Dohrenwend and B. P. Dohrenwend (Eds.), Stressful life events: Their nature and effects. New York: Wiley, 1974.

Egeland, B., Breitenbucher, M., and Rosenberg, D. Prospective study of the significance of life stress in the etiology of child abuse. J Consult Clin Psychol, 1980, 48, 195-205.

Endler, N. S. Person-situation interaction and anxiety. In I. L. Kutash et al. (Eds.), Handbook on stress and anxiety. San Francisco, Calif.: Jossey-Bass, 1980.

Friedman, M., and Rosenman, R. Association of specific overt behavior pattern with blood and cardiovascular findings. JAMA, 1959, 169, 1286-1296.

Friedman, M., and Rosenman, R. Type A behavior and your heart. New York: Knopf, 1974.

Gardner, R. A. Understanding children. New York: Aronson, 1973.

Garmezy, N. Competence and adaptation in adult schizophrenic patients and children at risk. In S. R. Dean (Ed.), Schizophrenia: The first ten Dean Award lectures. New York: MSS Information Corp., 1973.

Garmezy, N. Children under stress: Perspectives on antecedents and correlates of vulnerability and resistance to psychopathology. In A. I. Rabin et al. (Eds.), Further explorations in personality. New York: Wiley, 1981.

Garmezy, N., and Nuechterlein, K. H. Invulnerable children: The fact and fiction of competence and disadvantage. Am J Orthopsychiatry, 1972, 42, 328-329.

Gersten, J. C., Langner, T. S., Eisenberg, J. C., and Simcha-Fagan, O. An evaluation of the etiologic role of stressful life-change events in psychological disorders. J Health Soc Behav, 1977, 18, 228-244.

Gordon, D., Nowicki, S., and Wichern, F. Observed maternal and child behaviors in a dependency producing task as a function of children's locus of control orientation. Merrill-Palmer Quarterly, 1981, 27, 43-51.

Gottschalk, L. Vulnerability to "stress." Am J Psychother, 1983, 37, 5-23.

Holyrod, K. A., and Lazarus, R. S. Stress, coping, and somatic adaptation. In L. Goldberger and S. Breznitz

(Eds.), Handbook of stress: Theoretical and clinical aspects. New York: The Free Press, 1982.

Ilfeld, F. W. Age, stressors and psychosomatic disorders. Psychosomatics, 1980, 21, 56-64.

Jenkins, C. D. Psychosocial modifiers of response to stress. In J. E. Barrett (Ed.), Stress and mental disorder. New York: Raven Press, 1979.

Joe, V. C. Review of the internal-external control construct as a personality variable. Psychol Rep, 1971, 28, 619-640.

Kendall, P. C., and Hollon, S. D. (Eds.), Assessment strategies for cognitive-behavioral interventions. New York: Academic Press, 1980.

Kliman, G. W. Psychological emergencies of childhood. New York: Grune and Stratton, 1968.

Lefcourt, H. M. The functions of the illusions of control and freedom. Am Psychol, 1973, 28, 417-425.

Magnusson, D. Situational determinants of stress: An interactional perspective. In L. Goldberger and S. Breznitz (Eds.), Handbook of stress: Theoretical and clinical aspects. New York: The Free Press, 1982.

Mandler, G. Stress and thought processes. In L. Goldberger and S. Breznitz (Eds.), Handbook of stress: Theoretical and clinical aspects. New York: The Free Press, 1982.

Mednik, S. A., and Schulsinger, F. Studies of children at high risk for schizophrenia. In S. R. Dean (Ed.), Schizophrenia: The first ten Dean award lectures. New York: MSS Information Corp., 1973.

Miller, I. W., and Norman, W. H. Learned helplessness in humans: A review and attribution-theory model. Psychol Bull, 1979, 86, 93-118.

Minter, R. E., and Kimball, C. P. Life events, personality traits, and illness. In I. L. Kutash et al. (Eds.),

Handbook on stress and anxiety. San Francisco, Calif.: Jossey-Bass, 1980.

Moore, T. W. Stress in normal childhood. In L. Levi (Ed.), Society, stress and disease (Vol. 2). London: Oxford University Press, 1975.

Moos, R. H., and Billings, A. G. Conceptualizing and measuring coping resources and processes. In L. Goldberger and S. Breznitz (Eds.), Handbook of stress: Theoretical and classical aspects. New York: The Free Press, 1982.

Mullins, L. L., Siegel, L. J., and Hodges, K. K. Cognitive and life event correlates of depressive symptoms in children. Paper presented at the Annual Meeting of the American Psychological Association, Washington, 1982.

Myers, J., Lindenthal, J., and Pepper, M. P. Life events and psychiatric impairment. J Nerv Ment Dis, 1971, 152, 149-157.

Nowicki, S., and Strickland, B. R. A locus of control scale for children. J Consult Clin Psychol, 1973, 40, 148-154.

Pearlin, L. I., and Schooler, C. The structure of coping. J Health Soc Behav, 1978, 19, 2-21.

Phares, E. J. Locus of control in personality. Morristown, N.J.: General Learning Press, 1976.

Rabkin, J. G., and Struening, E. L. Life events, stress and illness. Science, 1976, 194, 1013-1020.

Rotter, J. B. Generalized expectancies for internal versus external control of reinforcement. Psychol Monogr, 1966, 80, (Whole No. 609).

Rotter, J. B. Some problems and misconceptions related to the construct of internal versus external control of reinforcement. J Consult Clin Psychol, 1975, 43, 56-67.

Rutter, M. Children of sick parents: An environmental and psychiatric study. London: Oxford University Press, 1966.

Rutter, M. Stress, coping and development: Some issues and some questions. J Child Psychol Psychiatry, 1981, 22, 323-356.

Rutter, M., Graham, P., and George, S. Temperamental characteristics as predictors of behavior disorders in children. Am J Orthopsychiatry, 1973, 43, 328-399.

Rutter, M., Maughan, B., Mortimore, P., Ouston, J., and Smith, A. Fifteen thousand hours: Secondary schools and their effects on children. Cambridge, Mass.: Harvard University Press, 1979.

Sarason, I. G., and Sarason, B. R. The importance of cognition and moderator variables in stress. In D. Magnusson (Ed.), Towards a psychology of situations: An interactional perspective. Hillside, N.Y.: Erlbaum, 1981.

Seligman, M. E. Helplessness: On depression, development, and death. San Francisco, Calif.: W. H. Freeman, 1975.

Shearman, K. An investigation into the relationships between maternal attitudes to the child aged 0-5 years, and some personality traits in the child at the age of eleven. Unpublished thesis, University of London, 1968.

Siegel, D. J. Separation-loss events, self concept, locus of control, and children's effective functioning in school. Unpublished doctoral dissertation, University of Pittsburgh, 1981.

Silber, E., Perry, S. E., and Bloch, D. A. Patterns of parent-child interaction in a disaster. Am J Psychiatry, 1957, 21, 159-167.

Solomon, Z., and Bromet, E. The role of social factors in affective disorder: An assessment of the vulnerability model of Brown and his colleagues. Psychol Med, 1982, 12, 123-130.

Sparacino, J. The type A behavior pattern: A critical assessment. J Human Stress, 1979, 5, 37-51.

Spivak, G., Platt, J. J., and Shure, M. B. The problem solving approach to adjustment. San Francisco, Calif.: Jossey-Bass, 1976.

Thomas, A., Chess, S., and Birch, J. Temperament and behavior disorders. New York: New York University Press, 1968.

White, R. W. Ego and reality in psychoanalytic theory. New York: International Universities Press, 1963.

Wills, T. A., and Langner, T. S. Socioeconomic status and stress. In I. L. Kutash et al. (Eds.), Handbook on stress and anxiety. San Francisco, Calif.: Jossey-Bass, 1980.

Yarrow, M. R. Child-rearing in families of working and non-working mothers. Sociometry, 1962, 25, 122-140.

Zautra, A., and Beier, E. The effects of life crisis on psychological adjustment. Am J Community Psychol, 1978, 6, 125-136.

5

BEHAVIORAL RESPONSES TO STRESS

The behavior that an individual manifests in response to stress may be viewed on a continuum from adaptive and relatively effective coping behaviors to the more extreme examples of ineffective efforts to meet the demands of stress. While a clear separation between effective and ineffective behavior is not always possible, such a distinction has often been drawn in the study of stress. The more successful efforts to cope have been seen as examples of adaptive behavior. Such coping responses have been studied in terms of problem-solving, competency, and mastery processes. They are typically seen as instances of active, goal-oriented effort, with some perceptual-cognitive element involved.

At the other extreme are the more clearly inadequate and inappropriate attempts to respond to stress. These are likely to be studied under the domain of psychopathology since they often result in behavior that is not only ineffective but often counterproductive, that is, against the individual's own best interests. If that individual is a child, such behavior may be seen as problematic by parents, teachers, and other adults. It has a negative impact on school work, peer relations, and the family. If the behavior comes to professional attention, it is likely to be labeled as a behavior disorder or an emotional adjustment reaction. Both ends of the continuum represent efforts to cope.

COPING RESPONSES

The theoretical formulations that have contributed to the study of coping have come from several sources. Psychoanalytic and ego psychologists have been led to adaptation and coping through the explorations of such ego functions as perception, language, memory, and thinking; processes that enable the individual to master and alter the environment (compare White, 1976). Haan (1977) reflects an ego psychologist's perspective in describing coping as an ego process that involves purpose, choices, flexibility, and adherence to consensual reality and logic.

Other theorists have taken a cognitive-behavioral approach, emphasizing the social learning and problem-solving aspects of coping (Kendall and Hollon, 1980). One of the better definitions of coping comes from Lazarus and Launier (1978, p. 311), who define it as "efforts, both action oriented and intrapsychic, to manage (that is, to master, tolerate, reduce, minimize) environmental and internal demands and conflicts among them which exceed a person's resources." They point out that the element of the definition referring to taxing demands limits the concept of coping to stressful situations rather than adaptation in general.

Several attempts have recently been made to identify the more common coping responses. Pearlin and Schooler (1978) designed a study to identify and compare the efficacy of coping responses of adult subjects. They viewed coping responses as what people <u>do</u> in their efforts to cope with life stress, thus making clear the distinction between them and coping resources. Through a series of interviews they sought to identify the coping repertoires individuals employed in dealing with stress in four role areas: marital, parental, household economics, and occupational. Thematic examination of interview material led to a series of questions reflecting coping patterns. The responses to those questions were then factor analyzed and a list of 17 coping responses was developed. While the authors acknowledge that the list represents only a portion of the coping responses available to adults, it is useful as an illustration of those responses typically employed. For example, those concerned with household economics were labeled as devaluation of money, optimistic faith, positive comparisons, and selective ignoring.

Pearlin and Schooler classified the responses they identified into three functional groups: (1) those which altered the situation generating the stress, (2) those which created more congenial perceptions of problematic experiences, and (3) those which function more in managing existing stress. The most common type of coping response is the second--those where the response functions to control the meaning of the situation. They refer to this as "cognitively neutralizing" the threat. Positive comparisons and selective ignoring are examples of this type.

In a promising effort toward identifying and classifying coping responses, Moos and Billings (1982) have proposed a preliminary taxonomy based on rational categorization. Their taxonomy divides nine common coping responses into three domains: (1) Appraisal-focused coping (logical analysis, cognitive redefinition, cognitive avoidance); (2) Problem-focused coping (seeking information or advice, taking problem-solving action, developing alternative rewards); and (3) Emotion-focused coping (affective regulation, resigned acceptance, emotional discharge). These categories are not mutually exclusive, nor do they exhaust the possibilities, but it is likely, as the authors contend, that they represent the major types of responses employed.

Some selected descriptions and examples provided by Moos and Billings (1982, pp. 218-219) will serve as good illustrations of the major coping responses:

> Logical Analysis. Strategies in this category include trying to identify the cause of the problem, paying attention to one aspect of the situation at a time, and mentally rehearsing possible actions and their consequences.
> Seeking Information or Advice. Responses in this category involve seeking more information about the situation; obtaining direction and guidance from an authority; talking with one's spouse, other relatives or friends about the problem; and asking someone to provide a specific kind of help, such as lending money.
> Affective Regulation. These strategies involve direct efforts to control the emotion aroused by the problem by consciously

> postponing paying attention to an impulse (suppression), experiencing and working through one's feelings, trying not to be bothered by conflicting feelings, maintaining a sense of pride and keeping a "stiff upper lip," and tolerating ambiguity by withholding immediate action.

Lazarus and his colleagues (Coyne and Lazarus, 1980) have emphasized the cognitive element in coping, which involves the appraisal of the event or situation. Their findings demonstrated that stressful events can be considerably more benign through cognitive means of achieving emotional control. Cognitive appraisal refers to the person's "continually reevaluated judgments about demands and constraints in ongoing transactions with the environment and his or her resources and options for managing them" (Coyne and Lazarus, 1980, p. 150). Cognitive appraisal, as can be seen from Lazarus' definition of coping given above, is an integral part of coping. This cognitive process is of crucial importance in discussing the coping efforts of children, who are limited by immature cognitive development.

While promising efforts, such as those advanced by Moos and Billings, have been made in identifying the coping responses adults commonly employ, children's coping responses have not been as systematically studied or organized. Rather, many of the efforts with children have focused on developing competencies to help them to cope more effectively (Cowen, 1982; Rubin, 1970). Although the responses employed by children might be expected to be similar to those found with adults, several factors serve to modify the responses and restrict the range of options available to children.

Children are limited in their responses by cognitive and language development, social maturity, and a lack of life experiences (previous learning) which results in fewer responses in their repertoires. Children lack the adult reasoning powers that come with maturity. Logical reasoning provides the justification for the tradeoffs, compromises, and balances that are necessary for adaptive living. Adults may also be capable of increased tolerance to stress, since reasoning helps them to see longer-term payoffs. Children have a more limited tolerance for frustration and for delay of gratification. Thus, developmental considerations serve to restrict the responses available to children.

Added to these developmental limitations are a number of other realistic restraints, such as a relative lack of mobility, financial and personal dependence on the family, home, and significant adults, all of which serve to limit their freedom to act in dealing with stress. An adult who finds himself in a stressful job situation may be able to modify his duties, change jobs, arrange for a transfer, resign, or relocate. The child who experiences school as a stressful situation may have few alternatives. Reducing stress by leaving the situation or consciously avoiding a potentially stressful situation are common strategies that require a certain degree of independence, planning, and mobility, which may not be available to the child.

MALADAPTIVE RESPONSES TO STRESS

Coping responses have varying degrees of effectiveness with some attempts clearly ineffective and even counterproductive. These are often socially unacceptable, extreme examples of coping behavior. In some cases they may be partially successful in meeting the demands of the primary stressor, but in the process, they create a new set of secondary stressors with which the individual will further have to cope.

Klerman (1979) sees adult depressive episodes as vain attempts on the part of the individual to adapt. Clinical depressions are, from his adaptational perspective, maladaptive outcomes of partially successful efforts at adaptation. In a similar way, childhood behavior disorders or emotional adjustment problems may also be seen as maladaptive responses to stress. In the case of children, the extreme responses that they adopt are manifested in behavior that calls attention to itself and interferes with effective functioning at home, in school, and in social relations.

While there is considerable variation in the ways individuals may respond to stress, depending on personality, social, and cultural factors, the range of human response is not infinite. Ultimately human nature restricts the options that are available to the individual and genetic factors and previous learning further limit them to a rather fixed repertoire for any one individual. As a result response patterns may follow a few basic themes, although there may be a number of variations on those themes.

Stress responses represent one type of human response to stimulus. In order to conceptualize them, a broader model of personality functioning is needed. Such a model would predict the major ways of responding to internal or external stimulus. A multidimensional, circumplex model has been developed to conceptualize human response. This model, depicted in Figure 5.1, employs two widely used dimensions of personality, active passive, and introversion-extraversion, which are related in an orthogonal configuration.

Man is a dynamic entity. He must reach out to interact with his environment in order to assure survival. Some degree of activity is always present. The infant, although greatly restricted in mobility, cries out and struggles in an effort to interact with the environment. Later, the child will slowly achieve a sense of mastery as he is able to affect objects and others in his world. Activity is a constant, and the degree of activity varies across individuals. Physiological studies have shown that the degree of activity is related to, among other things, the state of physiological arousal of the nervous system (Duffy, 1962). Activity serves as one of the underlying dimensions of personality.

The second dimension of personality reflects the direction toward which activity is expended. Some individuals tend to turn their activity toward the world. They are allocentric, outward-looking, and overtly active. These extraverts represent one end of a continuum, with the more introverted, withdrawn individuals at the other. Jung (1923) is often credited with having introduced this dimension to the study of personality, and it has become the most popular dimension utilized by personality theorists (Levy, 1970).

The vertical axis of the circumplex model describes the quantity of energy the individual expends, while the horizontal axis represents the direction of that activity, that is, turned outward toward the environment or inward toward the self.

It is possible to apply this general model of personality functioning to the more specific application of children's responses to stress. It is apparent from observations of children in schools and clinics that when children are under stress their activity levels vary. Some children tend to become overactive; some become lethargic and passive. Similarly, they may turn their activity inward, or

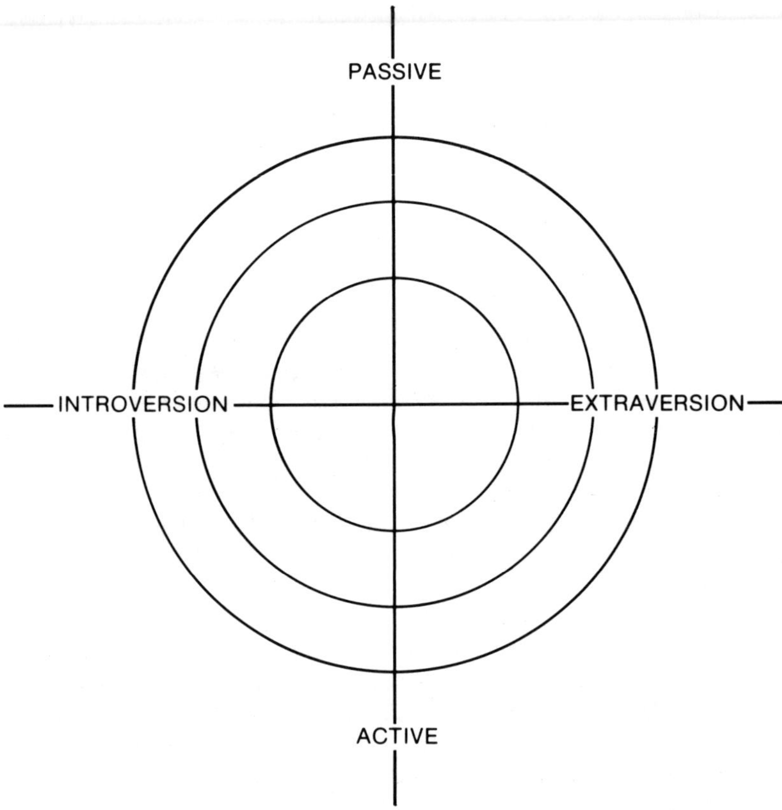

FIGURE 5.1

Two Dimensions of Personality

outward toward their environment. They may withdraw into quiet isolation or act out. These two basic dimensions, then, the active-passive and the introversion-extraversion, seem to be relevant in describing the behavioral responses of children to stress.

The model relates the two dimensions, illustrating how the response pattern a child might typically adopt in responding to stress can be seen on a continuum with extreme behavior at either end. In this context, the difference between normal functioning and the more extreme responses of the emotional adjustment reaction is one of degree. Emotional adjustment reactions, then, may be defined as extreme patterns of normal coping behavior adopted in response to stress (Figure 5.2).

The model yields four patterns of behavior, one for each quadrant. These can be seen as ideal types, in that they represent discrete, extreme cases of the behavior patterns. Figure 5.3 shows the four types of behavioral response patterns as they might apply to children.

As ideal types, they may be seldom found as discrete, isolated, and consistently predictable patterns in populations of children. Children's behavior varies widely, and they may adopt at times several patterns, although one usually tends to be preferred and may be seen as dominant. Clinical experience suggests that children showing these behavior patterns are commonly found in referred populations, and these patterns may be useful as diagnostic categories.

As diagnostic types they have been frequently found in the literature on child psychopathology (Clarizio and McCoy, 1978; Quay, 1979). Similar syndromes have also been occasionally identified through empirical studies (Edelbrock, 1979). A review of the literature and the psychological reports of children allowed characteristics for each type to be identified and collated so that composite descriptive statements could be developed (Chandler and Lundahl, 1983). The model, then, predicts four response patterns which may be seen as diagnostic types, and may be described as follows:

> The Dependent Child is often passive, immature, and characterized by regressive habits and childish mannerisms. This child lacks independence in many areas of functioning, and usually avoids taking the initiative in learning and social situations. Some children,

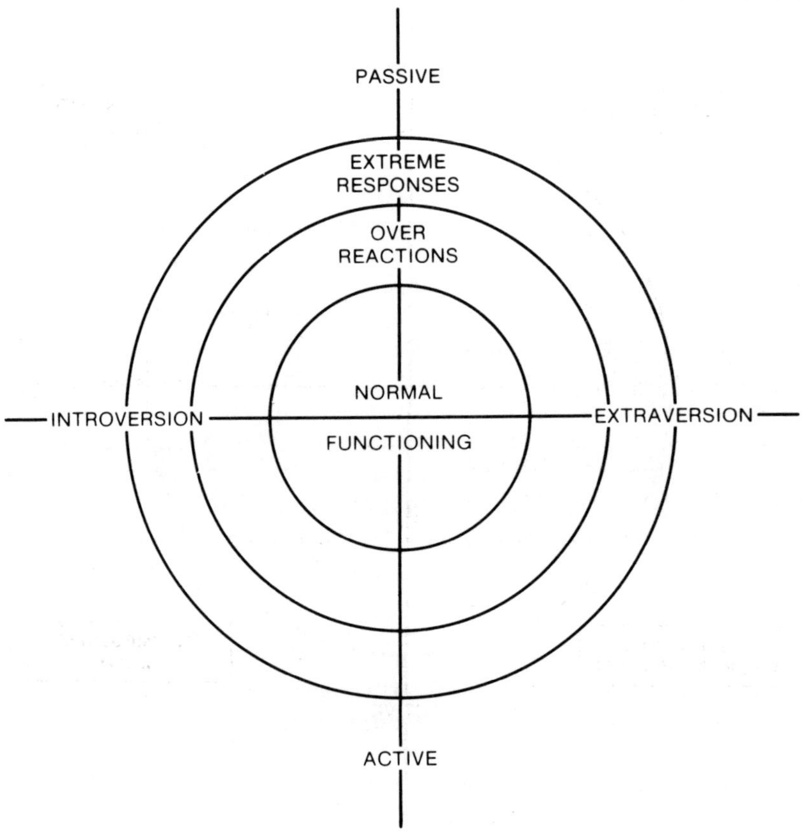

FIGURE 5.2

Degrees of Response

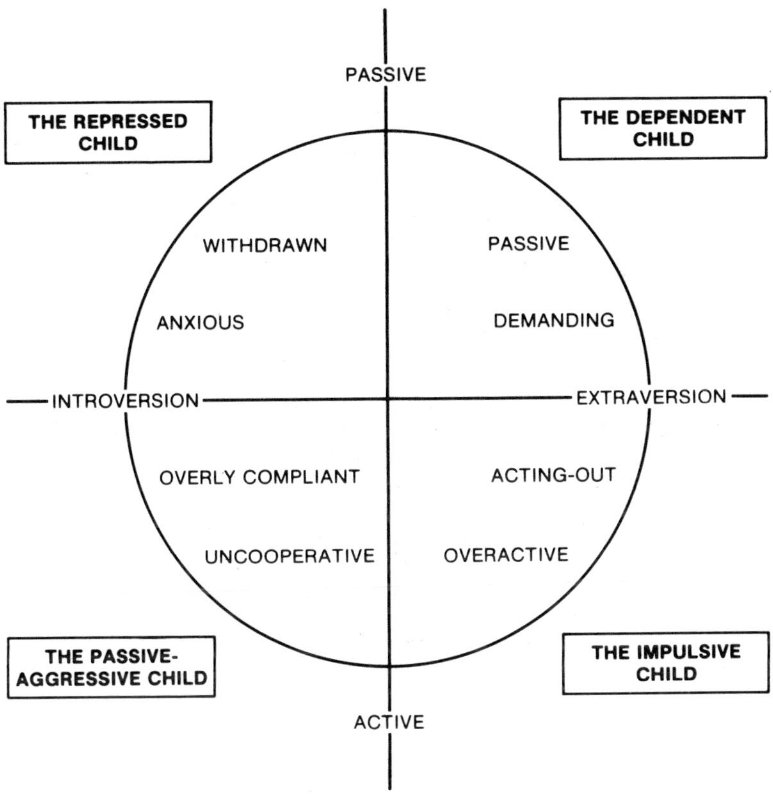

FIGURE 5.3

Four Common Response Patterns to Stress

while dependent, are less passive and adopt a more assertive, demanding manner to have their needs met. These children are often described as headstrong, defiant, selfish and willful. They seek immediate need gratification.

The Impulsive Child is easily excited, impulsive, and generally overactive. If the child's activity is focused, it may be turned toward authority figures or peers. Such children are described as aggressive and hostile, subject to temper tantrums, violence, and acting out behavior. For both subtypes, the essential problem is a lack of appropriate controls.

The Passive-Aggressive Child is most often characterized by school underachievement, and is usually described as indifferent about his poor grades in school. While sometimes these children adopt an obstinate, uncooperative attitude, others are overly compliant and agreeable, yet they fail to follow through on promises to complete assigned work, and they tend to procrastinate.

The Repressed Child is typically quiet, reserved, shy, moody, and detached. He seldom initiates conversation and is prone to daydreaming. Some of these children show symptoms of being anxious. This may involve fears, worries, nervous mannerisms, and overly sensitive reactions. They often have difficulty in making decisions.

If such maladaptive responses are distorted or extreme examples of common coping behaviors, it should be possible to relate them to identified coping responses. Table 5.1 provides an example of that relationship. It depicts four of the coping responses identified by Moos and Billings (1982) which might particularly apply to children, and matches them with what might be extreme instances of those coping responses, as predicted by the model.

Relating stress responses to a model of personality functioning suggests that such responses may act as personality traits, that is, they may become characteristic ways of responding employed in most situations. Such behavior patterns would constitute response styles.

Coyne and Lazarus (1980), in discussing coping models, note that a number of writers have pointed out that much of the observed consistency in human behavior can be related to individuals reacting in characteristic ways to their environment (Bandura, 1977; Bowers, 1973; Mischel, 1973; Runyan, 1978; Wachtel, 1973).

Table 5.1

Four Common Stress Response Patterns

Selected Coping Responses (From Moos and Billings, 1982)	Maladaptive Stress Responses of Children and Adolescents
Resigned acceptance. Accepting the situation as it is, with the feeling that nothing can be done to change things. Submitting to fate.	Dependent response. Such children seem resigned to being unable to effect change. They prefer to passively place their fates in the hands of adults.
Emotional discharge. Included here are verbal expression "to let off steam," crying, and impulsive acting out. May involve a failure of affect regulation.	Impulsive response. Such children are generally overactive and sometimes show aggressive, acting-out behavior. Their problem is one of appropriate control.
Developing alternative rewards. Attempts to deal with a problem by creating new sources of satisfaction. Developing greater autonomy and independence. Engaging in substitute pursuits.	Passive-aggressive response. Such children fail to meet adult demands, usually related to school performance. They stubbornly refuse to accept what they perceive as goals being imposed on them by others.
Cognitive avoidance. Denying fear or anxiety under stress, denial of the problem, engaging in wishful fantasies.	Repressed response. Such children show anxious, fearful, withdrawn behavior. They sometimes seem moody and detached.

Moos and Billings (1982) have suggested that hierarchies of coping preferences may characterize an individual during a life transition or life stage. In discussing the issue of stability, they cite evidence of considerable long-term stability in preferred ego-processes and cognitive style (Haan, 1977; Witkin and Goodenough, 1977), although they caution that the degree of cross-situational consistency of coping responses has yet to be determined.

The well-known investigations by Thomas and Chess (Thomas, Chess, and Birch, 1968; Thomas and Chess, 1977) into the temperament characteristics of children also provide evidence of the persistence of response styles. These authors maintained that the behavioral characteristics of children could be used to define personality types. They identified nine such behavior patterns or temperament categories based on their observations of babies and young children in their clinic: activity level, rhythmicity, approach/withdrawal, distractability, adaptability, attention span and persistence, intensity of reaction, threshold of responsiveness, and quality of mood. These characteristics were first seen in infancy and although they did not make a strong case for a genetic or constitutional base for temperament patterns, their work does lend some support to that notion (Lambert, 1982).

Finally, one might speculate that particularly with children who have been identified as having behavior disorders, there may be considerable cross-situational stability, since their persistent use of a preferred extreme response style may be a major reason why they have been identified and referred.

If coping responses in general, and maladaptive efforts in particular, can be shown to be relatively stable across situations, the partial taxonomy suggested by the model may be useful in classifying children who were referred because of functional emotional adjustment problems. A sample taxonomy, incorporating the stress response patterns, is presented in Figure 5.4.

Such a taxonomy has been in use at the University of Pittsburgh's Psychoeducational Clinic. A recent review of 100 consecutive cases of children seen for diagnostic psychological assessment found that over half could be classified according to their preferred response pattern (Table 5.2).

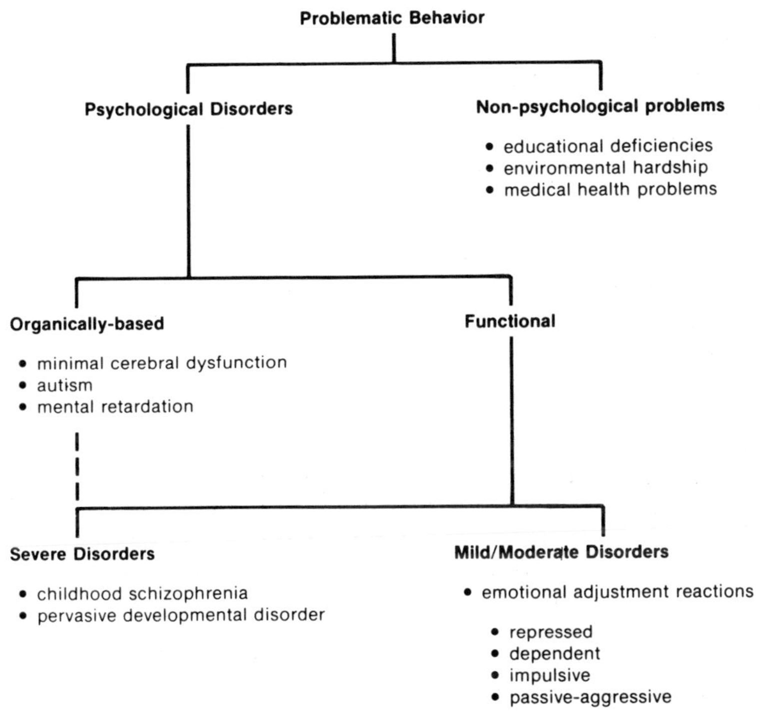

FIGURE 5.4

A Sample Taxonomy for Children's Behavior Disorders

TABLE 5.2

Diagnostic Classification of Cases Seen at the Psychoeducational Clinic
(n = 100)

Diagnostic Category		n
Mentally retarded		6
Learning disabled		4
Emotional adjustment reaction		56
Dependent	(11)	
Impulsive	(12)	
Passive-aggressive	(11)	
Repressed	(17)	
Mixed	(5)	
Other diagnosis		15
No significant problem		19

In order to test the reliability of the stress response classification scheme, the reports of the 56 cases that had been identified as those of emotional adjustment reactions were reviewed by an experienced psychologist familiar with the classification system as a result of a brief training orientation. This judge was given the descriptions derived for each category, as presented above, and asked to assign each case to one of the four categories, or to a fifth category designated as "mixed," that signified a mixture of behavioral symptoms. Agreement between case classifications was calculated by using Cohen's Kappa Coefficient, a measure of decision consistency useful with nominal data. Reliability was found to be good (K = .90).

Next, in order to further test the validity of the stress response classification scheme, an experimental instrument, the Stress Response Scale, was constructed by randomly assigning descriptors from each of the four response patterns to item positions in a six-point rating scale format. Items selected were those specific to neither home nor school environments so that both parents and teachers would be able to rate the child's behavior on a scale from zero to five: never, almost never, sometimes, often, almost always, always.

A series of developmental studies was then conducted using factor analysis on the scores derived from using the scale with various populations. One initial study (Chandler, 1979), employing a varimax rotated factor analysis of the scores using principle components, found a five-factor solution consonant with the classification scheme, which accounted for 62 percent of the variance. Replication with a modified version of the scale showed a similar factor structure, with a five-factor solution accounting for 70 percent of the variance (Piso, 1981). Moreover, the rating scales completed on both clinic-referred and nonreferred children had shown a similar factor structure, thus lending support to the contention that problem behavior may be seen as extreme examples of normal response styles. Since it had been shown that the behavior patterns of referred children were similar to those of nonreferred children, a subsequent study (Chandler and Lundahl, 1983) was designed to gather baseline data and further test the scale's validity with a sample of nonreferred children.

Subjects for this study were children ages five to 14 years, chosen randomly from rosters of kindergarten through eighth grade classes in two school districts in western Pennsylvania. Children in special education classes were excluded from the sample. Homeroom teachers at the targeted grade levels were asked to complete rating scales on three children in each class. The final sample was composed of 167 children: 82 boys and 85 girls.

Scores from the rating scales were subjected to a varimax rotated factor analysis using principle components. The clusters of items constituting the factors were then analyzed rationally to see if they would correspond to the predicted categories derived from the model.

Factors were drawn until Eigenvalues became less than 1.0. Five factors extracted met this criterion, and together accounted for 64 percent of the variance. An attempt was then made to define each factor and to compare the identified factors with the predicted diagnostic categories. Three of the four factors seem consistent with the diagnostic categories: passive-aggressive, repressed, and dependent. The fourth and fifth factors seemed to discriminate between the two subtypes predicted for the remaining category, impulsive. These were labeled as impulsive (acting out), and impulsive (overactive). Table 5.3 shows the symptom clusters identified by factor analysis.

TABLE 5.3

Symptom Clusters Identified by Factor Analysis

Impulsive (acting out)
Demanding (05)
Selfish (09)
Temper outbursts (11)
Defiant (17)
*Doesn't care about schoolwork (23)
Picks on other children (25)
Impulsive (26)
Willful (28)
Fights (29)
Detached, out of touch (34)
Headstrong (37)
*Unable to take criticism (38)
*Uncooperative (39)
Stubborn (40)

Impulsive (overactive)
Easily excited (03)
*Not quiet or withdrawn (08)
*Not passive (10)
Playful (19)
*Lack of participation (21)
Talkative (22)
*Not shy (30)
*Not afraid of new situations (35)
Headstrong

Dependent
*Not passive (10)
*Lack of participation (21)
*Lacks self-confidence (27)
*Not willful (28)
*Lacks independence (36)
*Unable to take criticism (38)

Passive-aggressive
Daydreams (02)
Underachiever (07)
Procrastinates, puts things off (13)
Poor attitude toward school (15)
*Lack of participation (21)
*Doesn't care about schoolwork (23)
Declining school grades (24)
*Lacks self-confidence (27)
*Doesn't complete assignments (31)
Detached, out of touch (34)
*Lacks independence (36)
*Uncooperative (39)
Stubborn (40)

Repressed
Worries (01)
Sensitive, easily hurt (18)
*Lacks self-confidence (27)
Nervous, jumpy (32)
Easily upset (33)
Afraid of new situations (35)

*Items with negative connotations have been reworded for this table in order to clarify their meaning.

In sum, factor analytic studies have supported the validity of the stress response scheme, and suggest that the behavior patterns often labeled as behavior disorders may be extreme examples of normal coping behaviors. From the analysis, the five syndromes identified as typical behavior patterns adopted by children are as follows:

Impulsive (acting out) children are often described as demanding, selfish, and defiant, with frequent temper outbursts. They are prone to fighting and picking on other children. They are impulsive, uncooperative, and stubborn, and have difficulty accepting criticism. They show a rather poor attitude toward school, usually not caring about schoolwork. They are sometimes mischievous, willful, and detached.

Passive-aggressive children are often described as underachievers who procrastinate, seem detached, daydream, tend not to complete assignments, show declining grades, and have a generally poor attitude toward school. They also tend to be uncooperative and stubborn.

Impulsive (overactive) children are often described as easily excited, mischievous, playful, and talkative. They tend to participate in activities and are not at all withdrawn, passive, or shy.

Repressed children are often described as being sensitive, easily hurt and upset, worrying, nervous, and lacking in self-confidence. They are often afraid of new situations.

Dependent children are often characterized as dependent and nonassertive. They lack self-confidence and are unable to take criticism. They seldom participate in activities.

SUMMARY

Children show behavioral responses to stress that range from the healthy, adaptive coping responses to those which are more extreme and maladaptive. Many of the coping responses available to, and commonly adopted by, adults are not available to children. Children are limited by developmental factors and reality restraints regarding the strategies they can employ in dealing with stress. The magnitude of their behavioral maladjustment may be seen as one indicator of the impact of stress.

Children who show emotional problems such as those labeled as behavior disorders or emotional adjustment reactions may be seen as manifesting maladaptive responses to stress. There is theoretical support and empirical evidence for a classification scheme that assigns children's maladaptive responses into one of four major response patterns: dependent, impulsive, passive-aggressive, or repressed. These patterns may be seen as diagnostic categories, and as such they may have implications for the assessment and treatment of children.

REFERENCES

Bandura, A. Social learning theory. Englewood Cliffs, N.J.: Prentice-Hall, 1977.

Bowers, K. S. Situationism in psychology: An analysis and a critique. Psychol Rev, 1973, 80, 307-336.

Chandler, L. A. A classification scheme for behavior disorders. Unpublished manuscript, University of Pittsburgh, 1979.

Chandler, L. A., and Lundahl, W. T. Empirical classification of emotional adjustment reactions. Am J Orthopsychiatry, 1983, 53, 460-467.

Clarizio, H. F., and McCoy, G. F. Behavior disorders of children. New York: Thomas Crowell Co., 1978.

Cowen, E. L. Primary prevention: Children and the schools. J Children Contemp Soc, 1982, 14, 57-68.

Coyne, J. C., and Lazarus, R. S. Cognitive style, stress perception, and coping. In I. L. Kutash et al. (Eds.), Handbook on stress and anxiety. San Francisco, Calif.: Jossey-Bass, 1980.

Duffy, E. Activation and behavior. New York: Wiley, 1962.

Edelbrock, C. S. Empirical classification of children's behavior disorders: Progress based on parent and teacher ratings. School Psychology Digest, 1979, 8, 355-369.

Haan, N. Coping and defending: Processes of self-environment organization. New York: Academic Press, 1977.

Jung, C. G. Psychological types. New York: Harcourt, Brace and World, 1923.

Kendall, P. C., and Hollon, S. D. (Eds.), Assessment strategies for cognitive-behavioral interventions. New York: Academic Press, 1980.

Klerman, G. L. Stress, adaptation, and affective disorders. In J. E. Barrett (Ed.), Stress and mental disorder. New York: Raven Press, 1979.

Lambert, N. Temperament profiles of hyperactive children. Am J Orthopsychiatry, 1982, 52, 458-467.

Lazarus, R. S., and Launier, R. Stress-related transactions between person and environment. In L. A. Pervin and M. Lewis (Eds.), Perspectives in interactional psychology. New York: Plenum, 1978.

Levy, L. H. Conceptions of personality. New York: Random House, 1970.

Mischel, W. Toward a cognitive social learning reconceptualization of personality. Psychol Rev, 1973, 80, 252-283.

Moos, R. H., and Billings, A. G. Conceptualizing and measuring coping resources and processes. In L. Goldberger and S. Breznitz (Eds.), Handbook of stress: Theoretical and clinical aspects. New York: The Free Press, 1982.

Pearlin, L. I., and Schooler, C. The structure of coping. J Health Soc Behav, 1978, 19, 2-21.

Piso, C. N. A revision, factor analysis and concurrent validation study of a children's behavior scale. Unpublished doctoral dissertation, University of Pittsburgh, 1981.

Quay, H. C. Classification. In H. C. Quay and J. S. Werry (Eds.), Psychopathological disorders of childhood (2nd Ed.). New York: Wiley, 1979.

Rubin, E. Z. A psychoeducational model for school mental health planning. Community Ment Health J, 1970, 6, 31-38.

Runyan, W. M. The life course as a theoretical orientation: Sequences of person-situation interaction. J Pers, 1978, 46, 569-593.

Thomas, A., Chess, S., and Birch, J. Temperament and behavior disorders. New York: New York University Press, 1968.

Thomas, A., and Chess, S. Temperament and development. New York: Brunner/Mazel, 1977.

Wachtel, P. Psychodynamics, behavior therapy, and the implacable experimenter: An inquiry into the consistency of personality. J Abnorm Psychol, 1973, 82, 323-334.

White, R. W. Strategies of adaptation: An attempt at systematic description. In R. H. Moos (Ed.), Human adaptation: Coping with life crises. Lexington, Mass.: Heath & Co., 1976.

Witkin, H. A., and Goodenough, D. R. Field dependence and interpersonal behavior. Psychol Bull, 1977, 84, 661-689.

6

THE STRESS ASSESSMENT SYSTEM

As we have seen, stress has been found to be associated with a wide range of psychological and physical problems of children. We have also seen the considerable impact it can have on their lives, especially if it is prolonged and severe. Because of interactive effects, stress often generates additional problems in living which, in themselves, become further sources of stress, thus establishing a vicious cycle.

As we have begun to better understand its role and the impact it may have on the lives of children, the relevance of an examination of stress in the assessment process becomes more compelling. Recently, the American Psychiatric Association recognized its importance when, in the most recent edition of its Diagnostics and Statistical Manual (DSM-III), it recommended that some survey of stressors be included as part of an assessment procedure (APA, 1980).

The study of stress suggests the need for an interactive paradigm which relates the various elements of the stress experience (Figure 6.1). The paradigm has direct implications for the assessment of children. The paradigm suggests that clinical assessment should be concerned with: (1) identifying the stressors in the child's life, that is, those events and situations which cause stress; (2) exploring the child's perceptions of those stressors; (3) assessing the impact of stress on the child's health, social, and school functioning, and (4) on his behavioral adjustment.

This chapter describes a multidimensional method, based on the stress paradigm being developed to systematically assess children's emotional status.

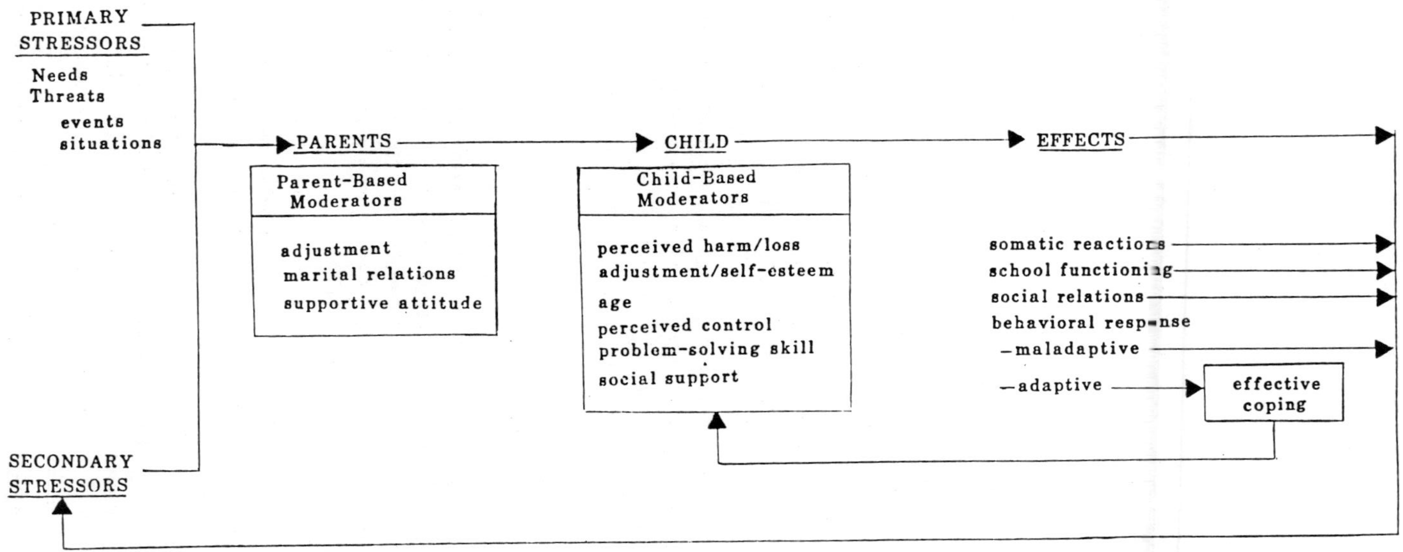

FIGURE 6.1

A Paradigm for Stress Analysis with Children

THE CHILDREN'S LIFE EVENTS INVENTORY

Rationale and Description

The interactive stress paradigm suggests that assessment should be concerned with identifying the sources of stress in the child's life. One class of stressors are those relatively discrete, short-term life changes that have been characterized as potentially stressful life events.

In order to survey the child's life for potentially stressful life events, some listing of commonly observed events in the lives of children is necessary. To be useful for clinical assessment purposes, such a listing should include events relevant to the family and home, and to the school, which are usually associated with some degree of distress. The Children's Life Events Inventory (CLEI) has been designed to meet this need.

The CLEI is a listing of 37 potentially stressful life events of children. These events have been arranged as items in a checklist format to be completed by parents (or other adults who are very familiar with the child's life history) during initial interviews. The adult is asked to check those events which have occurred in the life of the child. It takes approximately three to five minutes for most people to complete the inventory.

The Development of the CLEI

The CLEI is a modification of Coddington's list of life events of elementary school-aged children (Coddington, 1972). An examination of Coddington's list suggested that several aspects could be strengthened if the list were to be used in clinical assessment. Items which might normally not be seen as potentially threatening (for example, getting an award) were identified, since the CLEI would be constructed in accordance with a definition of stress which emphasized the perception of threat, rather than one which viewed stress simply as a disruption in equilibrium. These positive events were eliminated so that the resulting list would more clearly contain events associated with distress. Items of relatively low incidence (for example, discovery of being an adopted child) were also deleted since to be used clinically the list should be relatively concise with representative items. Inspection of Coddington's list also found relatively few school-related items, and so items were added that might reflect the stress associated with school and learning. In all, ten items from Coddington's original 36 were deleted and 11 added. The resulting list contained 37 events of elementary school-aged children usually associated with some degree of distress.

To test one aspect of the instrument's validity, a survey was conducted to see if mental health professionals and teachers would agree regarding the relative stressfulness of the events on the inventory (Chandler, 1981). Participants were asked to rate the events on the list in terms of relative severity on a scale from 0 to 20, assuming equal intervals, with the higher scores being the more stressful. The resulting mean scores were used to rank the events. Considerable agreement was found between these groups regarding the relative severity of the stress associated with each event.

Scoring and Interpretation

The CLEI provides a way of systematically surveying the histories and current life situations of children referred for clinical study. As such, it may help to identify those events which might be relevant stressors in the lives of children and to insure that significant events will not be overlooked in the assessment. In the process, it furthers the understanding of the child and can serve as a useful device in communicating with parents, teachers, and other professionals. Table 6.1 shows the incidence of CLEI items in a sample of normal children.

While the CLEI was originally designed to provide descriptive data, it is possible to quantify the data by a simple count of the number of events that have been checked. Used in this way, scores on the CLEI might be seen as estimating the level of risk or vulnerability. It might prove useful in screening processes where, along with other measures, it might help to estimate the range of risk for emotional disorders.

Finally, it is possible to compare children's scores against a normative group. Children might best be compared using the percentile ranks based on incidence scores as found in the CLEI manual. In this way, the child's percentile rank may be seen as another measure of estimated risk.

TABLE 6.1

The Incidence of Life Events of Elementary School-Aged Children (N = 407)

Item on CLEI	Number	Percent
Started school	407	100.0
Mother beginning work	223	54.7
Birth of brother or sister	207	50.8
Death of grandparent	182	44.7
Changed schools	163	40.0
Severe illness requiring hospitalization of parent	136	33.4
Loss of job by parent	136	33.4
Increased arguments with brothers and sisters	118	28.9
Family moves; relocations	107	26.2
Vision problem requiring glasses	102	25.0
Increase in number of arguments between parents	87	21.3
Marital separation of parents	81	19.9
Divorce of parents	78	19.1
Serious illness requiring hospitalization of child	76	18.6
Illness requiring hospitalization of brother or sister	69	16.9
Child needed special education services	66	16.2
Addition of a third party to family (i.e., grandmother)	66	16.2
Poor grades in school	65	15.9
Frequent absence of one or both parents	65	15.9
Speech problems	64	15.7
Learning problems in school	63	15.4
Increase in number of arguments with parents	58	14.2
Change in child's acceptance by peers	51	12.5
Brother or sister leaving home	47	11.5
Academic failure	40	9.8
Hearing problem	34	8.3
Marriage of parent to stepparent	25	6.1
Death of a close friend	25	6.1
Death of parent	23	5.6
Acquiring a visible deformity	8	1.9
Death of a brother or sister	8	1.9
Having a visible congenital deformity	6	1.4
Suspension from school	6	1.4
Jail sentence of parent	4	.9
Becoming involved in drugs and alcohol	2	.4
Foster home placement	1	.2

Summary of Research Findings

The CLEI has been used in a clinical setting for several years, and preliminary data have been collected. The research available on the CLEI to date has shown that:

1. Clinic-referred children, as a group, tend to have experienced significantly more SLEs than randomly selected children (Hoesch, 1982).
2. Age has been found to be an important variable affecting the number of events reported. As might be expected, older children, by virtue of having lived longer, will have experienced more SLEs than younger children (Hoesch and Chandler, 1983).
3. Socioeconomic status (SES) has been found to be another important variable affecting baseline data on the frequency of occurrence of SLEs in the lives of children. Research findings suggest that children from families in lower SES groups tend to have experienced significantly more SLEs than those from families in higher SES groups (Million, 1984).
4. The most appropriate method of scoring the CLEI may be a simple count of the number of events reported by the parents (Shermis and Chandler, 1984).
5. Baseline data, collected on the frequency of events on the CLEI in the lives of children, should be representative of various SES levels, and might best be organized by age groups. Such baseline data might prove useful in allowing the comparison of children when estimating the range of risk (Chandler, Million, and Shermis, 1984).

THE NEED-THREAT SCORING SYSTEM

Development and Description

One of the most important influences determining the magnitude of stress in a given situation is the individual's perception of that situation. There has been a general agreement in stress research that perception plays a vital role in mediating the effects of stress. Because of this crucial role, a stress assessment must be concerned with understanding the child's perception. Projective techniques seem especially suited to aid in that understanding, since they provide a method of ascertaining the meaning of a given situation, and thus estimating the relative stressfulness of that situation for the individual child. If such an analysis can be focused on the child's perception of unmet or partially met needs, as well as on perceptions of harm or loss associated with environmental demands, then some idea of the nature and severity of perceived stress can be gained.

A scoring system for the Children's Apperception Test (CAT), employing a need-threat analysis, provides a way of systematically analyzing a child's life stress situation. Various need-threat variables may be found in Murray's (1938) suggestions for interpreting thematic projective material. Murray advocated the analysis of Thematic Apperception Test stories in terms of the needs of the main character and the environmental forces to which he or she was exposed. Murray listed 44 needs and 20 press variables, a total of 64 variables that could be applied to each story.

Subsequent workers have modified Murray's scoring system. One promising modification was proposed by Cox and Sargent (1950). These authors developed a scoring method as a research tool for analyzing normative aspects of responses to selected TAT cards. In addition to needs and threats, Cox and Sargent analyzed the cards in terms of feelings, heroes, actions, and outcomes--six broad scoring categories with a number of variables in each.

The need-threat scoring system described here is an adaptation of the Cox and Sargent system. The original scoring categories were reduced, and needs and threats paired to form five need-threat binaries. When used as scoring categories, a sixth category, "other," is added to record the incidence of idiosyncratic responses or the simple enumeration of stimulus features of the card. Table 6.2 presents the need-threat binaries which are used as scoring categories.

Scoring and Interpretation

It is recommended that the CAT be administered to those children between five and nine years of age as part of the stress assessment.* In scoring the CAT protocol, the

*A similar scoring system is being developed for older children (ages ten through 14 years) using the Thematic Apperception Test.

clinician examines the responses to each card in terms of the five scoring categories, checking those which apply to each card.

TABLE 6.2

Need-Threat Scoring Categories

Independence-Domination. Need for freedom and autonomy; desire to resist domination, coercion; drive to rebel against authorities; desire for self-assertion. Feels coercion from others; loss of independence through domination by others, fear of losing freedom or being dominated.

Affiliation-Rejection. Need for forming relationships. Desire for friendship, love, acceptance, nurturance. Threat of being repulsed, ostracized, isolated or rebuffed; deprived of or denied affiliation, love, friendship, or acceptance by parents.

Security-Insecurity. Need for physical necessities (food, shelter, etc.); personal safety; protection from harm; fear of illness, death, catastrophe; danger in the environment, physical harm.

Achievement-Failure. Need for prestige, accomplishment, competence. Desire for success, recognition, respect, honor, power. Fear of inability to perform, failure, inadequacy, inferior status, lack of talent, prowess. Jealousy of the achievement of others. Fear of competition, rivalry.

Aggression-Punishment. Need to express hostility. Aggression directed toward peers and/or authority. Fears of punishment, violence from persons in the environment, being aggressed against.

Other. Unique or idiosyncratic themes. Enumeration of stimulus features.

Adding the number of checks for each scoring category and placing that number against the total number of checks for the entire protocol yields a relative percentage of responses for each category. This relative frequency of each category's occurrence in the child's protocol may be interpreted as an indicator of the relative significance of that binary as a source of perceived stress. This interpretation is consistent with the view that a frequently occurring element in a set of stories suggests particular meaning for the individual.

Summary of Research Findings

Research carried out on the need-threat scoring system to date has shown that:

1. A study of intra-judge reliability was conducted using four judges who were asked to score ten CAT protocols and, after a four-week interval, rescore the same ten protocols using the Need-Threat Scoring System. A mean rank order correlation of .78 was found for the four intra-judge pairs suggesting that individuals are fairly consistent in the way they score CAT protocols using the scoring system (Hughes, 1983).

2. A study of inter-judge reliability was conducted using four judges who were asked to score the same ten CAT protocols. The mean rank order correlation among the four judges was .69. In addition, the judges were found to generally agree as to the presence or absence of a specific binary, and they tended to agree regarding the primary and secondary need-threat binaries on the various protocols (Hughes, 1983).

3. In order to test an aspect of criterion-related validity, a study was conducted which compared the CAT protocols of clinic-referred and nonreferred children, both scored using the need-threat scoring system. The results found that clinic-referred children, as a group, showed significantly greater needs for security and threats of insecurity in their CAT protocols than did their nonreferred cohorts (Johnson, 1984). While these results are preliminary, and further research is indicated, they suggest that it may be possible to discriminate between clinic-referred and nonreferred children on the basis of their need-threat binary scores.

THE STRESS RESPONSE SCALE

Description

The development of the Stress Response Scale has been discussed in detail in Chapter 5. To recapitulate briefly, the scale was constructed of descriptors taken from the psychological reports of children which were thought to reflect the four behavioral patterns predicted by the stress response model. The conceptual model was then confirmed by a series of factor-analytic studies.

The current version of the scale has 40 items arranged on a six-point rating scale (0 = never to 5 = always). Rating scale items have been selected so that they can apply to either home or school environments, so that any adult familiar with the child's behavior (parent or teacher) can complete the scale.

The Stress Response Scale was developed as an instrument for use with children referred because of nonorganic, mild to moderate emotional problems. As such, it is not normally used with children with a primary diagnosis of mental retardation, psychoneurological learning disability, or severe emotional disturbance.

Scoring and Interpretation

The Stress Response Scale may be scored in two ways. First, a total score can be computed as an overall estimate of the severity of the behavior disorder. In addition, the total scores can be used to assign children to various ranges of risk based on their deviations from the normative group data. Used in this way the scale provides one measure of range of risk that can be used in combination with some of the other measures of the Stress Assessment System.

Second, subscale scores can be derived for each of the five response patterns: Impulsive (Acting Out), Passive-Aggressive, Impulsive (Overactive), Repressed, and Dependent. These scores may be plotted and a profile of the child's typical response pattern may be constructed. The profile may be seen as representing the typical behavior pattern the child is likely to adopt in responding to stress.

The assessment of the preferred stress response pattern has obvious implications for intervention. Guidelines based on what has been shown to be effective with similar behavior problems can be developed for the significant adults in the child's life. Intervention can then be directed at helping the child to adopt more realistic and effective means of coping.

The interpretation of profiles necessitates grouping the patterns according to some scheme. Clinical experience has suggested that profile scores of T $\geq$ 60 may have diagnostic significance. For convenience it is recommended that profiles be classified by two-letter codes, representing the two highest scores which exceed a T score of 60. (More complete rules for classifying profile patterns may be found in the SRS Manual.) Coding the profiles allows them to be classified and the resulting groups can be further analyzed to determine associated characteristics, and responsiveness to various interventions.

SRS data may be used in the assessment report in three ways: (1) by providing descriptions of the child's behavior; (2) by providing quantitative measure of the magnitude of the child's behavioral problem through the use of percentiles based on comparisons with the normative group data; and (3) by characterizing the severity of the behavior disorder or estimated range of risk, based on the normative data.

Summary of Research Findings

Research studies conducted with the Stress Response Scale have found that:

1. The Stress Response model has been shown to have both construct and content validity, and factor analysis provided further evidence of validity by confirming clusters of behavior consonant with the categories predicted by the model. The Stress Response model appears to be a valid representation of the behavior patterns children commonly adopt (Chandler and Lundahl, 1983).
2. Reliability studies with the scale using teachers as raters have yielded correlation coefficients of .80 and .86. Coefficient Alpha, a measure of internal consistency, was found to be .94 (Chandler, 1983).
3. Predictive validity was established by testing the scale's ability to discriminate between various groups of children. The Stress Response Scale consistently differentiated between clinic-referred and nonreferred children (Chandler, 1979; Piso, 1981; Chandler, 1983), and between children in regular education and those in special education programs for emotional maladjustment (Krotec, 1982).

4. Baseline data collected with children in regular education classes suggest that scores on the scale might best be interpreted by taking into account age and sex trends, and that ranges of risk may be established based on the total score (Chandler, 1983).

5. Cluster analysis of the scores of randomly selected children has identified several profiles of typical response patterns for boys and girls at various age levels. These data have implications for the clinical interpretation of stress response profiles (Chandler and Shermis, in press).

6. As a test of one aspect of criterion-related validity, Stress Response Scale profiles derived from the ratings of parents and teachers were compared with the psychiatric diagnoses assigned to children who had been referred for possible placement in special education classes for the emotionally disturbed. Evidence suggests that the scale may be sensitive to some of the psychiatric categories commonly assigned to children (Chandler, Shermis, and Marsh, 1985).

THE STRUCTURED PARENT INTERVIEW

Rationale and Description

In examining the effects of stress on the individual's life, Freud's dictum that a significant problem exists when it interferes with the individual's ability to love or work provides a useful guide. In the case of children, "love" might include social relations with parents, siblings, and peers, while "work" is clearly school functioning--the child analogue to adult work.

A third, and very important area, where the effects of stress have been widely studied, involves somatic symptoms. Psychophysiological research predates the more recent interests in the psychosocial aspects of stress, and role of stress in the etiology of various illnesses continues to be the subject of intense study.

Finally, in dealing with children, the effects of stress on developmental events might be especially crucial. So, a fourth area, development, would be a useful one to include in the assessment.

To assess the effects of stress on these important areas of functioning, some systematic procedure is needed for gathering data about the child's life, his history, and current situation.

Life history information has traditionally been gathered during a clinical interview intake or initial referral interview. Most interview procedures follow some logical guide or format. They may be loosely structured (for example, the open-ended questionnaire) or more highly structured (for example, checklists, rating scales). Generally, the more structured the interview, the more systematic data collection procedures will be, and as a result, standardization can be developed and reliability tested.

An estimate of the impact of stress must take into account its effects on the child's physical status, family and social relations, and school functioning. The Structured Parent Interview is an experimental instrument being developed to systematically survey those domains.

The interview elicits information on events, symptoms, and behaviors by questions arranged in a checklist format in four major sections. The first section is composed of seven questions dealing with early development. Since the relationship between disruptions in development and later susceptibility to stress is being increasingly recognized, data from this section may provide one measure of vulnerability to stress. The other three sections assess the effects of stress on: Medical/Somatic aspects (11 questions), School Functioning (eight questions), and Family/Social Relations (eight questions). These 34 questions are worded in such a way that a positive response indicates a possible problem.

Scoring and Interpretation

The instrument can provide descriptive and quantitative data. Used as a guide in structuring the interview, it can be helpful in understanding the effects of stress on the child's life. Counting the items checked as present in each area, as well as the overall total, provides quantitative data of potential value in establishing the reliability of the instrument, as in testing its validity by examining the ability of the scores to discriminate among groups of children.

The Development of the Structured Parent Interview

In developing the parent interview, a number of similar clinical interviews were reviewed (Dubus, 1984). Most interviews were found to be recommended procedures or semi-structured, open-ended instruments. However, regardless of the structure, some items seemed to recur with some frequency. A review of the literature on interviews (Dubus, 1984) and on the characteristics of children with emotional disorders (Kemmerer, 1984) also provided support for the items ultimately selected for inclusion.

Summary of the Research Findings

1. In order to establish validity by determining the relevance of the items to the life histories and current situations of children, a pilot study was conducted using the interview with parents of randomly selected samples of children. Age and sex were not found to be important variables affecting the total number of symptoms reported by parents. On the average, parents of randomly selected children reported 2.3 of the possible 34 items as problematic. Moreover, more than half of the parents indicated no problem, or one problem (out of the possible 34). These results provided some preliminary baseline data (Dubus, 1984).

2. In order to test the criterion-related validity of the interview, preliminary baseline data were compared with data from a sample of clinic-referred children. Initial results suggest that there may be differences in the total symptom count as reflected in the total raw scores of clinic-referred and nonreferred children (Kemmerer, 1984).

CLINICAL USE OF THE SYSTEM

The Stress Assessment System may have at least three clinical applications: as part of a screening procedure; in diagnostic classification; and in individual personality assessment. This section provides suggestions, and indicates directions that might be explored in using the system.

Screening Procedures

For some purposes it may be helpful to employ Stress Assessment System data in identifying children who might be particularly vulnerable to stress. Children at risk may be identified by several measures used in combination. For example, the child's percentile rank and range of risk on the CLEI can be seen as estimates of their vulnerability to stress. In a similar way, the developmental subscale of the Structured Parent Interview may be seen as another index of vulnerability.

Ranges of risk may also be established by using the total symptom count from the Structured Parent Interview, the magnitude of the behavior problem as derived from the SRS, and the relative frequency of stressful life events as measured by the CLEI. Figure 6.2 shows how the ranges of risk might be represented graphically.

While the Stress Assessment System may be useful as part of a screening battery, caution should be exercised in identifying children at risk. In this capacity, it should always be used in combination with other information. Further research is needed to establish the preferred methods of using the data, but preliminary findings suggest that it should be a potentially useful clinical method.

Diagnostic Classification

A comprehensive stress assessment must be multidimensional, providing information on several aspects of the individual's experience with stress. However, to move beyond an ideographic examination of the individual so as to be able to compare one child with another, some method of classifying children is necessary. While it may be useful for research purposes to classify children along any of the dimensions of the system, a promising approach for clinical study suggests classification by their behavioral response patterns.

One method of determining the response pattern to use in classifying the child is by means of the SRS profile. As has been pointed out, the SRS manual provides a procedure for classifying profiles by a two-letter code based on the two highest subscale T-scores to exceed 60. By collecting data on children who have shown similar profiles, it may be possible to collate associated features. A computer program has been developed to construct and analyze profiles by comparing them with data on children

THE STRESS ASSESSMENT SYSTEM FOR CHILDREN

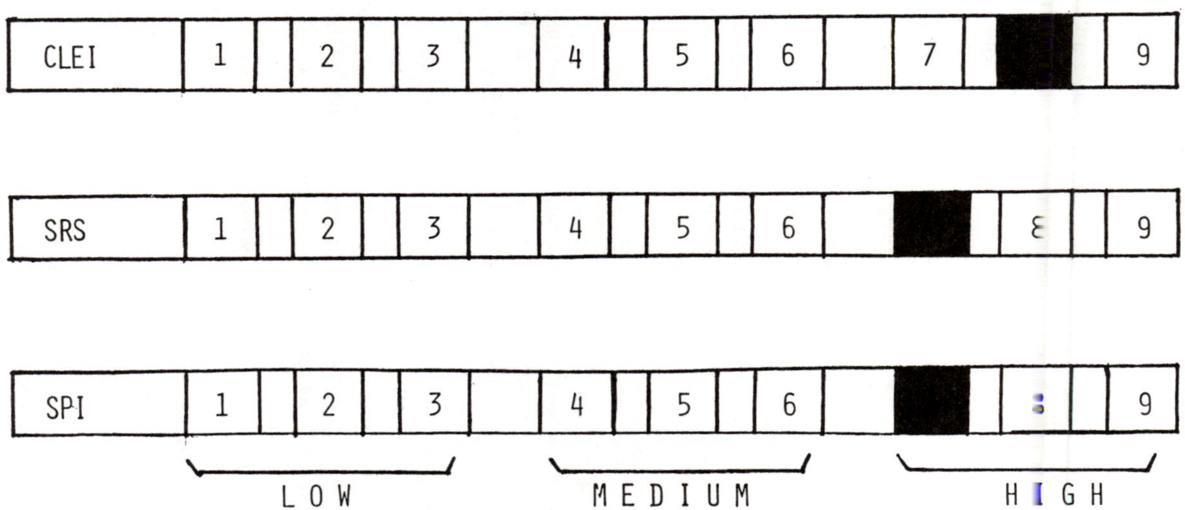

FIGURE 6.2

Severity Profile

seen for clinical services.* Figure 6.3 depicts a sample printout for the SRS Profile Analysis program.

Finally, some professionals may desire to select other diagnostic systems with which to work. There is evidence to suggest that SRS data might be useful in predicting assignment to some of the psychiatric categories commonly assigned to children from among those listed in the current edition of the Diagnostic and Statistical Manual of Mental Disorders (DSM-III) (Chandler, Shermis, and Marsh, 1985). Table 6.3 shows how SRS profile types may relate to selected psychiatric diagnoses. Further research is being conducted to examine concurrent and predictive validity with other typologies of childhood disorders.

Individual Personality Assessment

Once the nature of the problem has been identified, and is determined to be severe enough to warrant further professional attention, a more detailed examination is in order. At that point the other dimensions of the Stress Assessment System become relevant to understanding the child. Further information on the events and situations that may act as stressors, their timing during the child's development, the factors that lessen or exacerbate their impact, the level of the child's concern with various needs and threats, and the pervasiveness of the effects of stress are all areas that may require further exploration.

A psychological report, including a descriptive narrative of the child's life stress experience, might result from that analysis. Such a report would incorporate all three levels of the analysis by providing data on vulnerability and risk, the nature and severity of the problem, and a narrative description of the life stress experience. Examples of how a report might be organized are included in the Appendix.

---

*The SRS Profile Analysis Program is an experimental program. Inquiries from potential field test sites are welcome. Write to: The Psychoeducational Clinic, 5D Forbes Quadrangle, University of Pittsburgh, Pittsburgh, Pa. 15260.

SRS Results

Name:
Sex:
School/Clinic:

Date of Rating:
Child's age:
ID number:

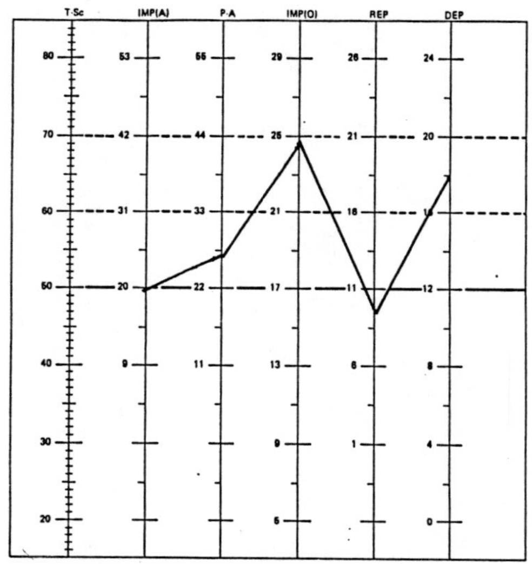

Subscale	Raw Score
Acting Out	20
Passive-Aggressive	25
Overactive	25
Repressed	09
Dependent	18
Total Raw Score	80
Total T-Score	56
Percentile:	85
Range of Risk	High
Profile type	DO/OD
Incidence of type:	
In normative sample	02%
In clinic sample	15%

Stress Response Descriptors: Unable to take criticism, lacks independence, active, playful, and headstrong. Associated Features: Within the clinical population this profile type is most commonly found with children with an average age of about 9 years. Such children show problems in school functioning most often described as inconsistent school work. There is likely to be evidence of psychosomatic symptoms (e.g., asthma, bedwetting, sleep and eating irregularities, headaches). Generally in test situations they are seen as showing adequate attention and concentration, but some anxious and dependent behavior is often manifested.

FIGURE 6.3 Sample SRS Profile Interpretation

TABLE 6.3

A Comparison of Selected SRS and DSM-III Diagnostic Categories

SRS Categories	DSM-III Categories
<u>Impulsive (Acting-Out)</u>. Acting-out children are often described as demanding, selfish, and defiant, with frequent temper outbursts. They are prone to fighting and picking on other children. They are impulsive, uncooperative, and stubborn; and they have difficulty accepting criticism. They tend to show a poor attitude toward school, usually not caring about schoolwork. They are mischievous, willful, and detached.	<u>Conduct Disorder, Aggressive Type</u>. The conduct disorder, aggressive child is often described as displaying persistent patterns of antisocial behavior that violates the rights of others. They are prone to bullying, physical aggression, and cruel behaviors toward peers. They may be hostile to adults, verbally abusive, impudent, defiant, and negativistic. Lying, truancy, and vandalism are common.
<u>Passive-Aggressive</u>. Passive-aggressive children are often seen as underachievers who procrastinate, put things off, have a poor attitude toward school, seem detached, daydream, don't care about schoolwork, tend not to complete assignments, and show declining school grades. They tend to be uncooperative and stubborn.	<u>Oppositional Disorder</u>. Oppositional children display pervasive opposition to all authorities, continual argumentativeness, and an unwillingness to respond to reasonable persuasion. Their oppositional patterns are generally passive and although they may appear to be conforming, they continually provoke adults or other children. They are negative and stubborn. They also procrastinate.
<u>Impulsive (Overactive)</u>. Overactive children are often described as easily excited, mischievous, playful, and talkative. They tend to participate in activities, and are not at all withdrawn, passive, or shy.	<u>Attention Deficit Disorder</u>. The ADD children are often described as impulsive, fidgety, restless, disruptive, and poorly organized. They exhibit excessive motor activity and have difficulty attending and paying attention. Their behavior is variable and functioning inconsistent.
<u>Repressed</u>. Repressed children are often described as sensitive, easily hurt, worrying, nervous, jumpy, easily upset, and lacking in self-confidence. They are often afraid of new situations.	<u>Anxiety Disorders</u>. Children with anxiety disorders are often described as irritable, overactive, lethargic, demanding of attention from adults, and generally unhappy. Their peer relations may be described as inhibited and they appear to be shy and fearful.

REFERENCES

American Psychiatric Association. Diagnostic and statistical manual of mental disorders (3rd ed.). Washington, D.C.: APA, 1980.

Chandler, L. A. A classification scheme for behavior disorders. Unpublished manuscript, University of Pittsburgh, 1979.

Chandler, L. A. The source of stress inventory. Psychology in the Schools, 1981, 18, 164-168.

Chandler, L. A. The Stress Response Scale: An instrument for use in assessing emotional adjustment reactions. School Psychology Review, 1983, 12, 260-265.

Chandler, L. A., and Lundahl, W. T. Empirical classification of emotional adjustment reactions. Am J Orthopsychiatry, 1983, 53, 460-467.

Chandler, L. A., Million, M. E., and Shermis, M. D. The incidence of stressful life events of elementary school-aged children. Unpublished paper, University of Pittsburgh, 1984.

Chandler, L. A., and Shermis, M. D. Assessing behavioral responses to stress. Educational and Psychological Measurement, in press.

Chandler, L. A., Shermis, M. D., and Marsh, J. The use of the Stress Response Scale in diagnostic assessment. J Psychoeducational Assessment, 1985, 3 (1).

Coddington, R. D. The significance of life events as etiological factors in the diseases of children. J Psychosom Res, 1972, 16, 7-18.

Cox, B., and Sargent, H. Brief reports, TAT responses of emotionally disturbed and emotionally stable children: Clinical judgements versus normative data. J Projective Techniques, 1950, 14, 60-74.

Dubus, J. T. Obtaining baseline data on children using a structured parent interview. Unpublished master's thesis, University of Pittsburgh, 1984.

Hoesch, A. H. Stressful life events of normal and clinic-referred children. Unpublished master's thesis, University of Pittsburgh, 1982.

Hoesch, A. H., and Chandler, L. A. Stressful life events of children: Implications for screening and assessment. Paper presented at the convention of the National Association of School Psychologists, Detroit, 1983.

Hughes, C. A. Reliability of a need-threat scoring system for projective material. Unpublished master's thesis, University of Pittsburgh, 1983.

Johnson, V. The use of a need-threat analysis of the Children's Apperception Test to discriminate between clinic-referred and non-referred children. Unpublished master's thesis, University of Pittsburgh, 1984.

Kemmerer, A. A comparison of the Stress Assessment data of clinic-referred and non-referred children. Unpublished master's project, University of Pittsburgh, 1984.

Krotec, S. C. A comparison of behavior, personality and academic variables of learning disabled, emotionally disturbed, and normal adolescents. Unpublished doctoral dissertation, University of Pittsburgh, 1982.

Million, M. E. Stressful life events of children: Their relationship to socioeconomic status. Unpublished master's thesis, University of Pittsburgh, 1984.

Murray, H. A. Explorations in personality. New York: Oxford University Press, 1938.

Piso, C. N. A revision, factor analysis and concurrent validation study of a children's behavior scale. Unpublished doctoral dissertation, University of Pittsburgh, 1981.

Shermis, M. D., and Chandler, L. A. Scoring a Children's Life Events Inventory: Weighted versus unweighted scores. Unpublished paper, University of Pittsburgh, 1984.

7

CHILDREN UNDER STRESS

This chapter presents some case material that has been selected to illustrate applications of the stress paradigm with children who have been referred for a variety of emotional and behavioral problems.

Cases have been organized by the diagnostic classification established by the stress response patterns. Wherever possible the significant sources of stress have been identified, and an attempt has been made to describe the child's perception of stressful events and situations. The result should be a case formulation with direct relevance for intervention and usefulness in understanding the child and communicating with parents, teachers, and other professionals.

The case of Alan is instructive because it shows how a child's perception of an earlier traumatic event continued to elicit a stress response some years later. Alan's maladaptive response to the perceived stress of that situation was seen in his impulsive, acting-out behavior.

Alan T.

Alan is an eight-year-old second grader who had been referred for clinical assessment because of angry outbursts in school. Alan seemed to show a very low frustration tolerance, and when corrected or criticized he was likely to respond with verbal outbursts or physical attack, often directed at peers or teachers. He frequently expressed the opinion that he was being "picked on."

Stress Assessment Results

An examination of the Children's Life Events Inventory showed that Alan had experienced only three potentially stressful life events. Two of those events were related: "vision problem requiring glasses," and "serious illness requiring hospitalization." (The third event, "beginning school," is common to all school-aged children.)

From a subsequent interview with his mother it was learned that Alan had developed a rather severe vision problem at age three resulting in a detached retina. At age three and a half he was hospitalized to have it re-attached. As a result, he currently has only peripheral vision in his right eye, and must wear protective lenses constantly. His mother reported that this had been an especially traumatic experience for Alan. The medical procedures and the separation from the family seemed to be especially stressful; and Alan seemed to understand that there was a possibility that he might lose his sight. He took quite a period of time to recover, later going through a period when he had frequent nightmares.

Alan's responses on the Children's Apperception Test showed that a significant source of stress for him was in his perception of the world as a threatening, punishing place. His stories describe aggression by larger (adult) animals against smaller (child-like) animals. There is a lion who uses his cane to hit and crush mice; and a hunter who pursues fleeing animals so he can kill them. In two stories animals are trapped underground in their burrows by threatening dominating figures. In one story, the conflict is clearly set between parents and their children. He tells of two little bears who have been fighting with their parents and are planning to run away. The immediate cause has been parental insistence that they go to bed, although they want to stay up to watch TV. In the end they are forced to go to bed, and they're feeling angry as a result. Still later, he tells the story of a little rabbit who is mad at his parents because they won't let him do what he wants. A needs-threat analysis identified the primary theme as the threat of aggression coupled with punishment and domination.

Alan's behavior, as profiled on the Stress Response Scale, shows him to have developed an impulsive response style. He tended to react angrily to criticism, was restless, overactive, and subject to temper tantrums.

Data from the Structured Parent Interview showed that he had a history of nightmares, although that was not a current problem. His other problems seemed largely confined to school functioning where they were seen by his parents as difficulties Alan was having in self-control.

Interpretation of Results

With this information it was possible to form some diagnostic impressions. It was hypothesized that Alan's barely repressed anger resulted from his perception of the hospitalization as a punishment inflicted on him by aggressive adults. He may have felt some lingering anger toward his parents for having "abandoned" him, and toward the medical personnel for the pain he suffered. In any event, he had clearly developed the view of others as punishing aggressors, and seemed likely to try counter-aggression as a way of defending himself against what he saw as arbitrary attack.

For Alan, the primary stressor was his visual problem and the resulting impairment. His misperceptions of that event led to several secondary sources of stress: his perception that he had been abandoned by his parents; his perception that he was being unfairly aggressed against by adults; and his own aggressive behavior adopted in response to stress.

Recommendations

It was recommended that counseling be considered for Alan and his parents. The objective would be to help Alan to better understand and cope with his visual problem, and to help him to change his perception of adult demands as threats. With his parents, efforts would be directed toward helping them to implement a reasonable discipline policy so that punishment would seem less aggressive to Alan. Finally, efforts could be made to modify Alan's impulsive behavior by a behavior management system so as to decrease his aggressive responses.

Michael A. manifested a common type of conduct disorder often associated with boys whose parents are going through a divorce. He, like Alan, can be seen as a child showing an acting-out, impulsive response pattern.

Michael A.

Michael is a seven-year-old who has a history of conduct problems which began in kindergarten. His second grade teacher has referred him for clinical assessment. He tends to be disruptive in class, with frequent temper tantrums, aggression toward peers, and generally impulsive behavior.

Stress Assessment Results

Of the four life events reported by Michael's mother, three related to marital problems. Those identified were: starting school, increased arguments between parents, frequent absence of one or both parents, and marital separation. An interview with Michael's mother confirmed that the last three years had been a difficult time for her marriage. There had been frequent arguments, with her husband occasionally leaving home. She and her husband were currently separated and had been discussing the possibility of divorce.

The picture which emerges from the Children's Apperception Test record was of a guilt-ridden child with numerous fears. Michael's stories were about animals who were fearful of the dark, and of strange noises in the night. In one story a rabbit is sitting in a crib, afraid to go to sleep because he believes in ghosts. In addition, a number of stories told of transgressions and inevitable punishments. A needs-threat analysis showed fears of punishment and insecurity to be two dominant concerns.

The Stress Response Scale profile showed an impulsive response style with both acting-out and overactive features. Michael was seen as a child who was unable to accept criticism, often defiant, fighting, and picking on other children. He was generally seen as active, impulsive, and easily excited.

On the Structured Parent Interview his mother reported that Michael had difficulty going to sleep, often resisting going to bed. He showed deteriorating functioning in school and in social relations with peers.

Interpretation of Results

Michael's impulsive behavior could be seen as a response to the stress associated with the marital troubles and separation, which was significantly impairing his functioning. It was hypothesized that Michael had strong feelings of guilt because he felt in some way responsible for the breakup of the marriage. He also seemed to fear punishment for his role, especially from his father. The stress resulting from his distorted perception of his life situation constituted a major problem for Michael, and his efforts to cope were ineffective and likely to cause further stress for him.

Recommendations

Because of the impact of the stress situation on Michael, professional treatment was recommended. Michael's mother could explore ways to reduce the overt stressors in his current situation through parent counseling. The management of sporadic visits from Michael's father, her own often unpredictable schedule, and competing demands on her time were all stress-related issues that could be discussed. In addition, psychological counseling was recommended for Michael to help him to gain a more realistic perception of the separation and impending divorce.

Brian represents another type of impulsive response—the overactive. With such children, their restless, distracted behavior and the resulting problems with attention create considerable problems in school functioning.

Brian Z.

Brian is a first grader who was having difficulty attending to schoolwork and accepting authority. His mother and his teacher referred him for clinical assessment because they were questioning his readiness for the second grade.

Stress Assessment Results

Brian's mother reported that he had experienced nine potentially stressful life events: beginning school, birth of sister, increase in number of arguments between parents, death of father, changed schools, academic failure, increased arguments with sister, increased arguments with mother, and foster home placement. From an interview with Brian's mother it was learned that Brian's father had died suddenly when Brian was three years old. His mother was subsequently hospitalized for mental illness, and Brian and his sister were placed in a series of foster homes. Midway through Brian's kindergarten year, the children returned to live with their mother. Brian changed schools after completing kindergarten, and was subsequently retained in first grade because his teacher did not feel he was ready to be promoted.

Brian's CAT responses were characterized by needs for nurturance, safety, and security. There were indications that he still had difficulty in coping with the death of his father. In one story a mother and her two children are returning from the store and spend the night in a house along the road. In the morning they return to their home, but their father is not there. By far the most powerful need-threat binary was security-insecurity.

Brian had developed an impulsive, overactive response style in response to stress. He was described as very restless and overactive, easily excited, easily distracted, and demanding.

An interview conducted with Brian's mother showed that Brian had shown a number of possible psychosomatic effects including numerous allergies and headaches. He was described as a picky eater. He had difficulty sleeping, was restless, and tended to wake up early. The other area of considerable impact was school functioning. He had been held back a grade, was considered to be an underachiever and a child who did not apply himself to his schoolwork.

Interpretation of Results

There appeared to be a direct relationship between the excessive number of stressful life events in Brian's history and his overactive behavior and consequent deteriorating school performance. It appeared that several major stressors including the death of his father, the hospitalization of his mother, and the foster home placements, all occurring within a relatively short period of time, had placed Brian under considerable stress. His poor school performance was creating still another set of stressors with which Brian and his mother would have to cope.

Recommendations

Because of the nature, severity, and pervasiveness of the problem, Brian's mother was referred for psychological counseling for herself and her child. It was felt that she would need considerable support and assistance in helping to manage and reduce the stress in their current life situation.

Donny was a child who had developed a dependent response style. His case also illustrates how the impact of a stressful life event will often be evident in thematic projective material.

Donny D.

Donny is a six-year-old first grader who attends a local parochial school. He has a history of bedwetting, and of generally immature behavior. Lately, he has been having problems in school coping with his work. His teachers describe him as a child who tries hard, although he had difficulty completing his work.

Stress Assessment Results

The Children's Life Events Inventory revealed that Donny had experienced four potentially stressful life events. In addition to starting school, they were: learning problems, academic failure, and the hospitalization of a sibling. The hospitalization had occurred following a fire in the home in which his older sister had been badly burned, when Donny was two years old. Subsequently, his parents had to spend an inordinate amount of time with his sister taking her for frequent treatments at the burn clinic.

Donny's responses on the Children's Apperception Test showed a significant source of stress in his perception of the threat of physical harm coupled with the strong need for security. In one story no one is home in the house. Two little babies are playing with each other, but they feel sad because no one is there, and they have been left all alone. In another story only a rabbit is at home and everyone else has left. He feels sad. He sees a door is open, and looks into the room to find the house is on fire. A needs-threat analysis indicated that Donny's major stress involved the need for security and the threat of insecurity.

A second source of stress was in his perception of the threat of parental domination.

Data from the Stress Response Scale showed that Donny had adopted a dependent style of responding to the stress he felt himself to be under. This included playful, demanding, stubborn, and generally immature behavior.

Finally, data from the Structured Parent Interview showed that Donny's problems were affecting his sleep habits (difficulty in falling asleep, bedwetting) and his school functioning.

Interpretation of the Results

The diagnostic description of Donny's problem may be formulated in the following manner. There are three major sources of stress for Donny: (1) his fears of physical harm and the threat of parental abandonment he associates with it; (2) the dependent style he has adopted in response to stress which, while partially successful in allowing him to regress to a less demanding level, has created further problems by increasing the ambivalence he feels toward his emerging drives for independence. As a result, Donny has become more extreme in his dependency, while, at the same time, resenting that dependency and fearing it will lead to a loss of independence; (3) the dependent response style has inhibited his initiative in school, and his childish resistance to domination has kept him from successfully completing school assignments, with the result that he is now experiencing academic difficulties which serve as an additional source of stress.

Recommendations

It was recommended that Donny be referred to a play therapy program in order to help him to express his fears and learn to cope with the threat of abandonment and harm. In addition, a behavior management program was suggested for Donny's parents to help them and his teachers to lessen his dependency and encourage more active, independent functioning at home and in school.

Like Donny, Judy showed a dependent response to stress, but her case also illustrates that, although a child with very few overt stressors in her history or current situation, she responds as though under stress.

Judy J.

Judy is a seven-year-old second grader who attends a local public school. She has been referred for clinical assessment by her teacher because of her concerns about Judy's excessive needs for social approval and peer friendship. She seems to be constantly seeking approval and reassurance, and her need for social stimulation is distracting her from her schoolwork.

Stress Assessment Results

A review of the Children's Life Events Inventory showed that, except for beginning school, there were no potentially stressful life events reported.

An analysis of Judy's thematic productions showed an intense concern with safety. There were dangers all around and a strong threat of being excluded from family or social groups. In one story a little girl is crying because she wants to go in, but those inside won't let her. The dominant need-threat binaries were affiliation-rejection and security-insecurity.

Judy's behavior pattern was characterized as dependent with helplessness, dependency, playfulness, and general immaturity.

An interview with Judy's parents indicated that there were problems in both school functioning and social relations. School problems were not considered too serious because Judy was able to maintain satisfactory grades in spite of her distractions. Social relations were affected, however, with her immature and clinging behavior causing her problems in making and keeping friends.

Interpretation of Results

The major source of stress for Judy is her perceived rejection by her parents and the accompanying fear of exclusion from her family. This has led her to adopt a regressive, immature response style in order to assure parental protection. Her inappropriate social behavior in constantly seeking approval and affection is a further effort to seek reassurance and meet her needs for security.

Recommendations

It was recommended that Judy be referred for psychological counseling through a program of expressive play therapy in order to help her to deal more effectively with her fears.

The next case represents a child who has developed a passive-aggressive response pattern. Like most children who adopt this response, his problem is not one of ability but one of willingness to work successfully in school.

Jason E.

Jason, a 12-year-old, was in the seventh grade when his parents brought him for clinical assessment. Jason's school work was declining. He appeared completely uninterested, was becoming argumentative, and seemed to have difficulty following instructions.

Stress Assessment Results

A review of the Children's Life Events Inventory identified 11 potentially stressful life events. Two important clusters had to do with family moves and relocations, and poor school performance. The former were related to Mr. E's work as an executive with a large national manufacturer. His position with the corporation required considerable travel, relocations, and at times the maintenance of two homes. The school-related events referred to a series of minor but increasingly significant school problems which began in the second grade.

In order to assess his perception of possibly stressful life events and situations, Jason was administered the Thematic Apperception Test. His protocol was characterized by parent-child conflicts. Four of the 12 stories told of conflict between parental and child wishes, usually resolved by the child being coerced into doing something. Story one is typical:

> In music class Johnny's teacher was giving demonstrations of different instruments, and he decided that he wanted to play the violin. So his parents got him a violin and he found out that he was faced with having to practice every night, and he didn't want

> to, but his parents made him. They locked him in his room to practice, but he just stared at the violin.

A needs-threat analysis of the protocol showed that the majority of the responses reflected the independence-domination binary.

Jason's behavior pattern on the Stress Response Scale suggested strong passive-aggressive qualities including being very independent and headstrong, declining school grades, procrastination, and a tendency not to complete school assignments.

Data from the Structured Parent Interview showed that physical complaints included a history of headaches often associated with difficult times in school. School functioning was marginal and inconsistent with an educational history that included tutors and special remedial help in reading. The general comment from Jason's parents and teachers was that he had good academic ability but didn't study or take an interest in schoolwork.

Interpretation of Results

Jason's poor school performance was seen as a result of a passive-aggressive behavioral style adopted in response to a perceived threat of parental domination and a strong need for independence. The perceived stress of his situation caused Jason to adopt a maladaptive response as a way of gaining control, asserting his independence, and resisting adult domination by simply refusing to apply himself to schoolwork.

Recommendations

Psychological counseling was recommended for Jason to help him to achieve a more realistic perception of academic demands. Counseling was also recommended for Jason's parents with the aim of altering their attitudes and behavior concerning their expectations and the demands they were placing on Jason.

Wilbur has developed a passive-aggressive response to life's stress situations. Like Jason, he showed obstinate oppositional characteristics that interfered with his effective functioning.

Wilbur T.

Wilbur, a 13-year-old eighth grader, was referred for psychological assessment because of a lack of motivation for schoolwork. He has been described as an underachiever, and he is currently failing in most of his coursework.

Stress Assessment Results

A survey of life events showed nine potentially significant events. In addition to beginning school, these were: death of grandparent, mother beginning to work, changing schools, family moves and relocations, learning problems in school, poor grades in school and academic failure, hearing problems and vision problem requiring glasses.

Wilbur's responses on the TAT contained frequent references to parental authority and conflicts between parent and child. In such conflicts the parent inevitably wins. A needs-threat analysis showed that, by far, the dominant binary was independence-domination.

Wilbur's stress response pattern showed strong passive-aggressive tendencies. He tended to procrastinate, was obstinate, headstrong, and demanding.

Data from an interview with Wilbur's parents showed that he had a medical history that included headaches, hearing problems, and vision problems. Wilbur has prescription eyeglasses but refuses to wear them. School functioning was also affected. He was seen as an underachiever who did not like school. No behavior problems were seen at school, but there were some difficulties reported in peer relations. Wilbur was described as a "loner," who had few friends. Because of his obstinate behavior, he was frequently in arguments with his parents. In sum, the effects of stress seemed pervasive in all areas of functioning.

Interpretation of Results

It was hypothesized that Wilbur had developed a passive-aggressive response style in reaction to what he perceived as unreasonable parental domination. In response to this perceived stress, Wilbur adopted strategies that were counterproductive to his own best interests.

Recommendations

Psychological counseling was recommended in order to help Wilbur to develop a more realistic perception of academic demands. In addition, counseling was also recommended for Wilbur's parents to help them to alter their attitudes and behavior regarding what they expected of Wilbur, and how those expectations were conveyed.

Paul's case illustrates that of a child who has developed a repressed response to stress, with overanxious and withdrawn behavior.

Paul B.

Paul, a 13-year-old eighth grader, had been referred for clinical assessment because of his mother's concern about his schoolwork. She reported that Paul had never worked up to his potential in school, but lately his attitude toward school was deteriorating, and he was failing all of his academic subjects. His teacher described him as lacking motivation and self-confidence.

Stress Assessment Results

The Children's Life Events Inventory showed that Paul had experienced a considerable number of potentially stressful life events including mother beginning to work, increase in number of arguments with siblings, change in acceptance by peers, academic failure, becoming involved with alcohol, learning problems, frequent absence of father, beginning school, child abuse, increase in number of arguments between parents, sister leaving home, poor grades, increase in arguments with parents, and drinking problems in the family. The number and severity of these events suggested a disruptive and possibly chaotic family life as a major source of stress.

Paul was administered the Thematic Apperception Test, and his responses reflected a violent and chaotic world view. There were themes of death with people being attacked, dying, or often fleeing, running away, and otherwise leaving horrible situations. He described one picture as a young man who died from a disease. An older man is blessing the body. He then added that many more would die of the same disease. A needs-threat analysis showed strong needs for affiliation with fears of rejection, punishment, and aggression.

An analysis of the Stress Response Scale showed that Paul tended to adopt repressed behavior in response to stress. He worried excessively, was nervous and jumpy, and often seemed detached and out of touch.

Data from the Structured Parent Interview showed that Paul's physical status had been affected (he had difficulty sleeping at night). His relations with family and friends had also been affected. But by far the greatest impact had been on his school functioning. These results suggested that the effects of stress were severe and pervasive.

Interpretation of Results

Paul was seen to be under considerable stress from a number of environmental stressors. He was unable to cope with his chaotic, disruptive family life, and was showing deteriorating school performance and interpersonal relations.

Recommendations

There was a clear and immediate need to introduce some stability into Paul's home life. Once this initial step was accomplished, subsequent efforts could be made to help Paul to cope more effectively.

Like Paul, Robby has developed a repressed stress response. The high level of anxiety and related symptoms bear some resemblance to adult neurotic conditions.

Robby S.

Robby is a seven-year-old student in the first grade at a local public school. Because of parental concerns about his excessive shyness and his manifest anxiety, especially seen when he has to take tests in school, Robby's parents have referred him for clinical assessment.

Stress Assessment Results

The Children's Life Events Inventory showed seven potentially stressful life events. Along with beginning school these included: birth of sibling, loss of job by parent, family moves and relocations, severe illness requiring hospitalization of parent, frequent absence of one or both parents, and learning problems in school.

Robby's CAT protocol was characterized by themes of accidents and injuries occurring to youngsters while parents are absent or unresponsive to the dire consequences. Of particular importance was absence of the father, usually associated with some disaster, while his presence offered protection. Five of the ten cards elicited themes in which a child has difficulty falling asleep, and the father's presence is comforting. A needs-threat analysis showed that by far, the dominant binary was security-insecurity.

The Stress Response Scale showed many behavioral manifestations of an anxious, repressed response style, including excessive worrying, shyness, and nervous, jumpy behavior. There were also indications of dependent tendencies.

A Structured Parent Interview showed that Robby had difficulty sleeping at night. School functioning seemed relatively unaffected with the important exception of test taking, which seemed to be especially difficult for him.

Interpretation of Results

Robby's overanxious repressed response was seen in reaction to perceived stress arising from a threatening environment where he might be left unprotected. There were a number of stressful events that might have contributed to these perceptions, including the hospitalization of the father, his losing his job, and his frequent absences.

Recommendations

In order to help him to cope more effectively with his fears, Robby was referred for psychological counseling. The objective would be to help him to gain a more realistic perception of environmental threats and the necessity of parental protection against perceived harm.

8

INTERVENTION WITH CHILDREN

Relating the emotional problems of children to stress raises some obvious implications for treatment. These implications may be formulated as a set of questions that might prove helpful in guiding intervention:

1. Is it possible to reduce stress through environmental manipulation?
2. Is it possible to reduce stress through changing the attitudes and behavior of significant adults?
3. Is it possible to modify the child's extreme behavior so that it more closely approximates normal coping responses?
4. Is it possible to reduce stress by helping the child to adopt a more realistic perception of himself and his life situation?
5. Is it possible to reduce the effects of stress by training in stress management techniques?
6. Can stress, the child's response to it, and/or its effects, be modified by some combination of the above?

These questions should be considered sequentially since the initial ones are more likely to be the preferred approach for most children. The first two, or possibly the first three, may not involve the child in direct contact with a professional. Direct intervention with a child carries with it some identification and labeling, and the fact that the child has been singled out for intervention is likely to result in an additional source of stress. A guiding principle should be: direct intervention should be undertaken only when indirect methods are not feasible, or likely to be ineffective. Indirect intervention, most often employing parents (or teachers) as agents of change, has several features that recommend it.

SIGNIFICANT ADULTS AS AGENTS OF CHANGE

The child's world is largely shaped by the significant adults around him. Children are dependent on adults not only for their economic care and physical well-being, but also for the quality of the emotional climate in which they must live and grow. Adults act as powerful models for the young and impart a view of reality that is of considerable influence during the child's formative years.

In general, adults guide children, helping them in their development to adjust to increasing reality demands. Reasonable adults do not seek to insulate the child from those demands, but they do provide some cushioning of the harsher aspects of reality. Adults, then, serve as mediators, filtering and interpreting reality for children.

The crucial role parents play in interpreting stressful life events provides a good example of adults as mediators (see Chapter 4). It has been shown that parents help to order and structure a stressful situation, thus assisting the child in understanding and integrating the experience.

In addition to their active roles as mediators, adults can provide an environment in which children can experiment, learn, and grow. They can try to ensure that that environment is not unduly stressful.

Environmental stress in the home and family or in the classroom can be reduced by imposing some order, structure, and predictability on the environment. Clear adult expectations and effective communication are also helpful. These environmental qualities lessen childish fears, decrease ambiguity, and generally reduce the sources of potential stress inherent in day-to-day living. By creating a low-stress home environment, parents provide a secure base from which the child can venture forth to meet the more stressful reality demands of the neighborhood and the school.

Teachers, too, can reduce the inevitable stress of school on youngsters (Chandler, 1981). Teachers who accept their roles as responsible adults, who impose reasonable control and discipline on the classroom, and who make their expectations for academic performance clear, reduce ambiguity, minimize the opportunities for frustration, and lessen anxiety and insecurity in the children in their classrooms. Coming to terms with academic demands is the central task of the child in school. The stress associated with it, and the opportunity it presents to develop effective coping resources, should be the single most important concern. Other stressors, such as those created by a confusing, chaotic, or fearful environment, should be eliminated or minimized.

Adults in general, and parents in particular, because of their powerful influences as models, mediators, and environmental manipulators, can be potent forces for change in working with children. Adults are invested with magical powers by the very young, and some vestige of that perception lingers throughout the developmental years (and probably into adulthood). The adult is for the child the person in charge, bringing order out of chaos, correcting wrongs, balancing the injustices, and controlling the forces that, if left unchecked, might prove overwhelming. Children therefore tend to see adults as protective and helping.

Because of the immense power of parents, many professionals who work with children prefer, if possible, to enlist the active support of the parents in the intervention process (Simpson and Poplin, 1981). It has been clearly demonstrated that the most effective intervention programs are those where the parents were able to understand and support the professional's efforts (Allen and Harris, 1966; Berkowitz and Graziano, 1972).

METHODS OF TREATMENT

Counseling with Parents and Their Children

Counseling with parents and their children has a diversified heritage reflecting the influence of a number of theoretical sources. Psychoanalytic insights, cognitive-behavioral principles, issues in human development and social learning contributions have all influenced the practice of psychological counseling. While each of these contributions may have something relevant to offer in any individual case, the result has often been an eclectic, pragmatic approach employing a variety of methods and techniques.

In addition to theoretical differences, there are differences in the manner in which such counseling is conducted. Five configurations are possible: child-centered individual counseling; parent-centered counseling; collateral parent-child counseling; family counseling; or some combination of these various configurations. The configuration selected might be determined by a number of factors including theoretical orientation, the understanding of the nature and severity of the problem, and the differences between adults and children as clients.

A number of writers have commented on the latter consideration as an important determiner affecting how counseling can be carried out (White and Watt, 1973). Certain limits are imposed on the process when the client is a child. Clarizio and McCoy (1976) suggest that motivation for treatment, insight into treatment objectives, linguistic development, dependence on environmental forces, and plasticity of personality are all differences between adults and children that have implications for counseling.

Despite differences in theory and practice, some common conceptual ground may be possible if a stress paradigm is employed in understanding the problem. Furthermore, if counseling is related to a stress assessment process, the implications of the assessment can clarify the objectives and assist in selecting the methods for counseling.

Of all the varieties of psychological counseling and psychotherapeutic methods, the techniques developed within the framework of brief, short-term therapy seem especially suited to the stress paradigm. Brief therapy has four fundamental elements (Rosenthal, 1980): time-limited duration--usually from three hours to as long as six months; a focus on specific issues; a "here and now" orientation; and a family-focused approach, which, in the case of children, means primarily the parents. Barten and Barten (1973) have described the method as an active, focused, incisive intervention communicated to child, parent, or both. They have further pointed out that since the attitudes and behavior of significant adults are often instrumental in initiating and maintaining problem behavior on the child's part, it is frequently more effective to work with adults as major participants in brief therapy.

Ronny G.*: A Case Study

Ronny, a seven-year-old, was brought to the clinic by his mother because of her concern about his personality development. She described him as "two different boys," one passive, obedient, and quiet; one overactive, loud, and a behavior problem. She saw the most dramatic shift in his behavior when he was under the care of his maternal grandmother. At these times, particularly, he became overly dependent and demanding, frequently asking for help, and reverting to more immature speech and language. In addition, he was having problems in school. His grades were declining, and he frequently complained about a lack of friends. He was having trouble meeting the academic and social demands of the first grade to such a point that the teacher was considering retaining him for a year because of his immaturity.

Ronny's mother had been divorced since he was five, and, since she worked full time, he spent a great deal of time in the care of his grandmother. Mrs. G. was concerned about the influence her mother was having on Ronny because she felt her mother tended to be too permissive and overprotective. There were differences of opinion between mother and grandmother about child-rearing, and specific disagreements about his eating habits. Ronny was mildly overweight, and his mother was concerned about his tendency to put on weight. His grandmother tended to minimize the issue, and would covertly encourage Ronny to have snacks behind his mother's back.

Psychological assessment found Ronny to be an insecure child who had adopted a dependent response style as a manner of reacting to perceived stress associated with the divorce and his uncertainty about his subsequent status with his mother. The uncertainty was exacerbated by his mother's rather irregular work schedule. He reacted to the resulting stress by regressing and assuming the role of a much younger child, a role his grandmother readily allowed him to assume.

At the initial session, the therapist was able to confirm Mrs. G's suspicions that her son was developing

---

*This case was presented as part of a larger article by the author which appeared in Psychology in the Schools, 1983, 20, 215-218, and which is used here by permission.

some dependent personality traits, and her role and her mother's role in that development were clarified. While his grandmother reinforced the regressive behavior by satisfying his every whim, Mrs. G. was able to demand and receive more appropriate behavior. This suggested that Ronny was capable of acting responsibly when adult expectations were made clear. He was confused by the contradictory messages from the two significant adults in his life, and sought to manipulate the situation.

The goal of therapy was to change the attitudes and behavior of significant adults so as to modify Ronny's maladaptive (dependent) responses to stress. In the process one major source of stress, the ambiguity arising from differing adult expectations, would be addressed initially. In order to achieve the goal several objectives were identified: (a) change the behavior of Ronny's grandmother and/or lessen her influence; (b) develop some consistency in the approach taken by significant adults by reinforcing responsible, age-appropriate behavior; (c) demand a consistent level of performance in his schoolwork, reinforcing him for work well done; (d) better monitor Ronny's weight.

While it proved difficult for Mrs. G. to change Ronny's grandmother's attitude toward him, it was possible to reduce the time he spent with her, thus lessening her influence. Changes that Mrs. G. had instituted to lessen her mother's influence also caused some confrontations between the two adults, giving her the opportunity to make her desires clear. Once her position was established, Ronny's grandmother's behavior began to change, and, with the greater consistency shown by the adults in his life, Ronny's behavior also improved.

The second and third goals were related, and work on them depended initially on Mrs. G. recognizing and verbally reinforcing Ronny for any evidence of more responsible behavior. For example, it was recommended that she no longer keep reminding him to get ready for school in the morning. It was made clear to him that that was his responsibility. After a few days of uncertainty, Ronny was able to be more or less ready to meet his bus on his own. Mrs. G. then praised him by telling him that she was proud of his efforts.

Since school was becoming an increasingly important source of stress, the therapist also contacted the teacher. The problem of contradictory messages from significant adults was discussed, and her help was solicited. She was asked to take a similar approach, for example, demand more responsible behavior. Poor, messy schoolwork was to be quietly returned to him with the single comment, "I know you can do better than this." The message given was to be that substandard work simply would not be accepted. On the other hand, special effort was made to praise good work in school.

Finally, Ronny's weight was considered as a major source of stress. His mother was given a height/weight chart with a graph of the normal growth curve for boys plotted on it. This chart was placed above the bathroom scale, Ronny would be periodically weighed, and his weight plotted on the chart. Mrs. G. reported that this technique had an immediate effect on Ronny's efforts to control his weight, which had been the cause of much of the teasing at school and contributed to his feelings that he had no friends.

There were weekly sessions with Mrs. G. during the six-week brief therapy period. The most immediate and dramatic change had to do with Ronny's attitude toward his weight problem. He became actively involved in the effort to reduce and hold his weight down. Changes were also noticed by his teacher. His schoolwork began to improve, and he became more involved in the social life of the classroom. He began to develop some friends. There was less whining, demanding behavior at home, and as relations between parent and child improved, Ronny seemed to be much happier. His school work continued to improve to the point where the teacher felt confident in recommending that he be promoted to the second grade.

A brief therapy, as a problem-solving process focusing on the sources of and responses to stress, can be effective in bringing about significant change for a child and his parents.

STRESS MANAGEMENT STRATEGIES

Neuromuscular Relaxation

Because of the interactive effect of physiological and psychological changes, stress management techniques that focus on lowering physiological arousal levels have received considerable attention. Suinn and Deffenbacher

(1980) list a number of methods used to acquire relaxation including relaxation training, hypnosis, autogenic training, breathing exercises, meditation, and biofeedback. Two techniques will be discussed here because of their promise in the treatment of stress-related disorders: relaxation training and biofeedback.

Jacobsen (1938, 1939) is generally credited with being the first to advocate a technique for learning to relax certain muscle groups. He showed that pulse rate and blood pressure could be diminished by deep muscle relaxation. His progressive relaxation technique involved getting patients to tense muscles and then to be aware of their experiences as they released that tension. By concentrating on various muscle groups, such as shoulders and neck, eyes, and chest, patients could become aware of the experience of relaxation. Once aware of the experience, Jacobsen proposed that they could acquire conscious relaxation through further training and practice.

Since the work of Jacobsen, relaxation has been shown to have a calming effect, modifying many of the indicators associated with the physiological stress response. Muscle relaxation has been found to reduce heart rate, respiratory rate, and skin conductance (Paul, 1969).

Benson (1975) has advocated a technique that combines elements of relaxation and meditation. The aim is to develop a relaxation response which decreases and counteracts the increased activity of the sympathetic nervous system associated with the physiological stress response. He maintains that the regular practice of the relaxation response can lower blood pressure, heart beat, respiratory rate, and oxygen consumption, all indicators that increase when the subject is under stress. He sees the regular practice of the relaxation response as useful in managing the stress endemic in day-to-day living.

Richardson, Beall, and Jessup (1982) have demonstrated how adolescents can be trained in progressive relaxation. They included a stress management unit as part of a school health education program. They found that high school students could be taught relaxation techniques in 15 50-minute class periods over three weeks. They also found that training in muscle relaxation and related methods produced a measurable reduction in heart rates, and they concluded that stress management training might be made a regular part of the school health program.

There have been a number of programs developed to extend the training of relaxation to children (Humphrey, 1984; Lupin, Braud, Braud, and Duer, 1976; Stroebel and Stroebel, 1984). Day and Sendak (1982) reported on one study using Benson's relaxation techniques with groups of elementary-school children. Subjects in a treatment group practiced relaxation each morning for ten minutes over a six-week period, while a control group was given instruction in reading. Results indicated that the subjects in the treatment group scored lower on a general anxiety scale and also on a test anxiety scale than did a control group. However, a follow-up study, conducted three weeks after the termination, showed that the treatment effects had disappeared. While such efforts may be promising, further work is necessary to better understand the usefulness and limitations of the application of relaxation techniques with children.

One of the more promising advances in the development of relaxation techniques has come from the pairing of relaxation training with biofeedback. Biofeedback instruments are devices which, when connected to subjects, measure and display physiological functions, usually in the form of light or sound signals. The subject then tries to change the function in a desired direction by cognitive or subjective states. Since changes in function are immediately known, the subject is able to alter his efforts until, by trial and error, he learns to control that function (Patel, 1981).

Interest in biofeedback grew from studies that demonstrated that techniques of operant conditioning could be used to control functions of the autonomic nervous system generally assumed to be outside of the individual's control (Miller, 1969, 1978). The rationale behind the procedure is that a knowledge of success reinforces the learning. A major practical consequence of the developments in biofeedback has been the demonstration of the clinical usefulness of relaxation training (Stoyva and Anderson, 1982).

While there is some disagreement regarding whether biofeedback-assisted relaxation is superior to simple verbally induced relaxation (Nuechterlein and Holyrod, 1980), biofeedback does offer some practical advantages. It provides the sort of immediate reinforcement that may be of considerable value in motivating further effort (Stoyva and Anderson, 1982).

Amar (1980) has detailed a biofeedback training program for clinical use with children. She maintains that children seem to learn physiologic control rapidly, and thus are excellent candidates for biofeedback training. There are other advantages to using this technique with children. For example, the electronic feedback monitors and equipment can be made appealing to children as a sort of electronic "game" so that the child's cooperation and motivation can be maintained.

In the procedure recommended by Amar, the therapist sits with the child, demonstrating the equipment, then modeling the skill to be learned, and finally coaching the child in the training. She feels that children relate naturally to the therapist in the role of coach, since they easily become involved in the game and skill-learning aspects of the task.

The child is then asked to sit quietly and watch the light display. Initially changes can be reinforced by some material reinforcer, for example, a small toy, although later material reinforcers can be quickly phased out.

In a clinical therapy situation Amar recommends a typical course of biofeedback training to last about 24 sessions, that is, 12 weeks of twice-weekly one-hour sessions. Follow-up sessions may have to be scheduled as needed. Amar reports on a case of an 11-year-old girl who had been referred with a history of migraine headaches. She was taught Jacobsen's technique of progressive relaxation paired with biofeedback electromyographic training on a twice-weekly basis. After eight weeks of training there was a significant decrease in symptoms and the girl's mother reported that she seemed happier and less tense.

While relaxation training is often coupled with biofeedback, it is also found in tandem with systematic desensitization.

Systematic Desensitization

In systematic desensitization, a physiological state that is inhibiting of anxiety is induced by means of muscle relaxation (Wolpe, 1982). The subject is then exposed to a mildly stressful stimulus for a few seconds. As the process is repeated, the severity of stress associated with the stimulus begins to lessen. It is then possible to introduce stimuli that are similar to the original, but potentially more stressful to the subject. Stimuli can be arranged on a hierarchy of severity of stress as gradually more stressful stimuli are introduced. The basis of desensitization, the gradual exposure to fearful situations by degrees, has long been a technique used by parents to help their children to overcome their fears.

Wolpe (1958, 1982), who is often credited with developing and popularizing this technique, acknowledges a debt to Jacobsen's work on progressive relaxation. He saw the possibilities in applying Jacobsen's techniques in treating his patients who were in psychotherapy for various anxiety disorders. He began by linking a gradual exposure to phobic stimuli with an active, anxiety-inhibiting response on the patient's part, the relaxation response.

The method Wolpe advocates is composed of four phases: (1) the introduction of a subjective anxiety scale, (2) training in deep muscle relaxation, (3) the construction of anxiety hierarchies, and (4) counterposing of relaxation and anxiety-evoking stimuli from the hierarchies (Wolpe, 1982, p. 141). He cites evidence for the efficacy of this technique in treating phobic disorders.

A recent example of a study of systematic desensitization was provided by Kipper and Giladi (1978). These investigators applied the technique to a group of college students who were having difficulties with test anxiety. First, subjects were taught relaxation techniques. Next, an anxiety hierarchy was constructed. Items were arranged in a progressive order, from least to most anxiety evoking, culminating in an actual test situation in a classroom. The relaxation response was elicited as the subject was exposed to each item on the hierarchy. The study provided evidence that systematic desensitization could be effective in reducing the stressfulness of test situations.

Research over 20 years on desensitization therapy supports the conclusion that it has had a significant impact on anxiety responses associated with specific stimuli (compare Suinn and Deffenbacher, 1980).

Cognitive-Behavioral Techniques

The cognitive-behavioral approach to intervention covers a wide range of treatment procedures including cognitive restructuring, modeling, and behavioral and imaginal rehearsal. In general this approach recognizes the importance of cognitive mediators in the elicitation and maintenance of anxiety. From this viewpoint it is not so much the stimulus itself that elicits the anxiety as it is the personal constructs or meanings that the person brings to the situation (Beck, 1976). This suggests that if positive change is to occur, cognitive aspects may have to be changed accordingly.

Suinn and Deffenbacher (1980) describe the rationale for a therapy based on cognitive restructuring this way:

> If distorted cognitive patterns prompt anxiety, then it follows that changing these belief systems to be more rational and socially appropriate should tend to decrease affective arousal, defensive avoidance and disrupted performance. Viewing the world in more reasonable terms may leave the individual experiencing frustration and other mildly negative emotional states but should free the person to engage in whatever problem-solving and cognitive behaviors are at his disposal. This is exactly the goal of cognitive-restructuring approaches; for example, for clients to develop more reasonable appraisals of themselves and the world (p. 406).

An example of a cognitive-behavioral technique that incorporates several stress management strategies is the stress inoculation procedure outlined by Novaco (1979). Novaco extended the stress inoculation concept that was originally proposed by Meichenbaum (1975), for the treatment of anxiety, to the treatment of anger.

Novaco sees anger as an affective stress reaction. It can be adaptive if it leads to assertive, coping behavior, or it can be maladaptive if it prompts impulsive, aggressive action. Novaco's coping skills therapy for the treatment of anger has, as its aim, minimizing the maladaptive effects and maximizing the adaptive functions of anger.

The procedure moves through three phases: cognitive preparation, skill acquisition, and application training. It employs elements of relaxation training, assertiveness training, recognition of arousal, self-monitoring and instructing, the learning of coping skills, and problem solving. Novaco (1979) has presented evidence for the usefulness and effectiveness of these procedures with various client populations.

Much of the work extending cognitive-behavioral methods to the treatment of children has been influenced by Meichenbaum (1979). Cognitive-behavioral studies with children initially focused on the problem of impulse control. Meichenbaum (1979), reviewing a number of studies, concludes that self-control can be established in children by methods employing self-instruction training, modeling, rehearsal, prompts, feedback, and social reinforcement.

Meichenbaum has done much to popularize the use of self-instruction training as a cognitive-behavioral technique useful with children. He views self-instruction as a method which supplements the normal developmental process of acquiring self-regulation. He notes that the "private speech" many children employ as a self-regulatory device is an interim stage in the developmental process. The original source of direction and control of the child's behavior is the speech of the care-taking adult (Meichenbaum and Goodman, 1971). Eventually overt speech is internalized to become inner speech or thoughts that regulate behavior. Since impulsive children have failed to develop the necessary behavioral control, it seems reasonable to assist them by using verbalizations.

Consistent with the position outlined by Meichenbaum, Douglas (1972) has advocated training techniques to teach children to "stop, look, and listen." One such training procedure has been demonstrated by Palkes, Stewart, and Kahana (1968). Palkes et al. constructed 5 x 7 cards as reminders for children about to engage in academic tasks. The cards bore such reminders as "stop," "listen," and "look and think before I answer." The child was to verbalize the self-directive commands before attempting each task. If the child failed to verbalize the command, the experimenter would point to the relevant card and insist that the child state the command before proceeding. Subsequent use of the command was reinforced by a positive comment by the experimenter. Substantial improvement was seen in work performance after children had had a number of rehearsals of the self-instructive statements.

While the initial studies of the use of cognitive-behavioral techniques were concerned with impulsive children, a number of other applications have been forthcoming. Once cognitive-behavioral methods had been shown to be effective in developing self-control in children, attempts were made to extend their use to academic tasks (Meichenbaum and Asarnow, 1979). Meichenbaum and Asarnow (1979) advocate self-instructional methods to improve reading, mathematical skills, and memory recall. Most of these employ some combination of cognitive modeling and rehearsal procedures designed to teach children strategies of what to say prior to performing some task.

Meichenbaum and Asarnow offer evidence regarding the effectiveness of cognitive-behavioral procedures applied to academic functioning. They cite the work of Douglas et al. (1976), who studied the effects of modeling, self-verbalization, and self-reinforcing techniques on hyperactive boys. They found improvement on a variety of cognitive and motor tasks, such as listening, spelling, and oral comprehension tests for children who had undergone cognitive training.

Cognitive behavioral methods seem to hold considerable promise as means of assisting children in stress management. However, a cautionary note seems in order. Johnson (1982) discusses a number of techniques such as modeling and rehearsal used to prepare children for potentially stressful events. She is particularly concerned about the use of stress management as a preventive measure. She points out that techniques sometimes employed as preventive may actually increase a child's anxiety by calling attention to potential problems, and she urges caution in applying stress management techniques with children.

FURTHER CONSIDERATIONS

Before leaving the topic of intervention with children, two further considerations deserve discussion. The first is drug therapy. In this context, the use of medication is viewed as a supportive therapy. In some cases it may facilitate relaxation, helping the child to be more receptive to other forms of stress management.

Generally, three types of drugs have been commonly used with children showing behavior problems: (1) CNS stimulants, useful in treating the hyperkinetic syndrome; (2) antipsychotics, for the treatment of severe emotional disorders; and (3) minor tranquilizers (anxiolytics) and sedatives, often used in treating anxiety in adults and in treating children who show nervous, anxious, fearful behavior and sleep disturbance.

The third type of drugs may prove to have particular relevance for children under stress; however, Conners and Werry (1979) warn that there are almost no data on the usefulness of those drugs beyond clinical impressions. They point out that sedatives and anxiolytics have not been well studied in children, although they may have some limited usefulness. They further speculate that some of the absence of data may be due to the fact that anxiety is highly placebo sensitive (Conners, Eisenberg, and Sharpe, 1965; Eisenberg, Gilbert, Cytryn, and Molling, 1961).

The finding that there is a strong placebo effect present in the treatment of anxiety leads to the second consideration, that is, the nonspecific aspects of the treatment of stress. Whenever professional help is solicited, the possibility is raised that some placebo effect may be, at least in part, responsible for therapeutic change. Rosenthal and Frank (1956), in applying the placebo concept from medicine to psychology, maintain that any credible procedure applied in a socially sanctioned manner is likely to result in some improvement. Such professionally applied treatment methods may be efficacious regardless of the specific technique employed, especially when procedures are new and their proponents enthusiastic (Frank, 1961).

Nonspecific placebo factors may be defined as those common to most types of therapy. These include suggestion, persuasion, treatment credibility, therapist attention, expectancy of cure, and demand for improvement (Critelli and Neumann, 1984). Fish (1973) has detailed a treatment based on the explicit recognition of the nonspecific aspects of therapy. He suggests that the therapist carefully formulate a believable placebo consistent with the client's belief structure. The therapist then engages in a healing ritual which persuades the client that it is what he does, rather than what the therapist does, that results in the cure.

The possibility that placebo factors may be particularly important in stress management, especially with those techniques that rely heavily on technology, has been raised by a number of workers (Amar, 1980; Bowers and Kelly, 1979; Gaardner and Montgomery, 1977). Gaardner and Montgomery (1977) discuss the placebo effect in the context of biofeedback training. They see biofeedback techniques henbaum, D. A self-instructional approach to stress management: A proposal for stress inoculation training. In C. Spielberger and I. Sarason (Eds.), Stress and anxiety (Vol. 2). New York: Wiley, 1975.

ichenbaum, D. Cognitive-behavioral modification: Future directions. In P. Sjoden et al. (Eds.), Trends in behavior therapy. New York: Academic Press, 1979.

eichenbaum, D., and Asarnow, J. Cognitive-behavioral modification and metacognitive development: Implications for the classroom. In P. Kendall and S. Hollon (Eds.), Cognitive-behavioral interventions: Theory, research and procedures. New York: Academic Press, 1979.

Meichenbaum, D., and Goodman, J. Training impulsive children to talk to themselves: A means of developing self control. J Abnorm Psychol, 1971, 77, 115-126.

Miller, N. E. Learning of visceral and glandular responses. Science, 1969, 163, 434-445.

Miller, N. E. Biofeedback and visceral learning. Annu Rev Psychol, 1978, 29, 373-404.

Novaco, R. The cognitive regulation of anger and stress. In P. Kendall and S. Hollon (Eds.), Cognitive-behavioral interventions: Theory, research and procedures. New York: Academic Press, 1979.

Nuechterlein, K. H., and Holyrod, J. C. Biofeedback in the treatment of tension headache. Arch Gen Psychiatry, 1980, 37, 866-873.

Palkes, H., Stewart, M., and Kahana, B. Porteus Maze performance of hyperactive boys after training in self-directed verbal commands. Child Dev, 1968, 39, 817-829.

Patel, C. H. Yoga and biofeedback in the management of hypertension. In D. Wheatley (Ed.), Stress and the heart. New York: Raven Press, 1981.

as sharing, along with such elements of the therapeutic relationship as the patient's faith and wish to trust, some responsibility for the efficacy of treatment. Suggestion and ritual are two elements of the placebo effect which, they maintain, have considerable potential within themselves.

Bowers and Kelly (1979) have provided evidence for the role of suggestion and hypnotic susceptibility in the psychological treatment of stress-related disorders. They argue that even in those interventions that are not explicitly hypnotic, suggestion and hypnotic susceptibility may be hidden factors that promote healing.

Their discussion of psychotherapy in relation to stress-induced disorders is worth reviewing here. Bowers and Kelly conceptualize the psychotherapeutic attempts to treat psychosomatic disorders along a continuum of specificity. Least specific are the conventional psychotherapies that have as their aim better psychological functioning. Next are those techniques that focus on reducing stress by lessening the threatening characteristics of the environment or increasing the patient's resources to cope more effectively. Finally, they consider the most specific therapies to be those that focus on ameliorating or eliminating some particular somatic dysfunction. They see biofeedback and relaxation techniques as being in this group. With those methods, and with many of the other techniques designed to assist in stress management, suggestion and the client's susceptibility to hypnosis seem to be common elements.

REFERENCES

Allen, K., and Harris, F. Elimination of a child's excessive scratching by training the mother in reinforcement procedures. Behav Res Ther, 1966, 4, 79-84.

Amar, P. B. Application of biofeedback training in children. In G. P. Sholevar et al. (Eds.), Emotional disorders in children and adolescents. New York: Spectrum, 1980.

Barten, H. H., and Barten, S. S. (Eds.). Children and their parents in brief therapy. New York: Behavioral Publications, 1973.

Beck, A. T. Cognitive therapy and emotional disorders. New York: International Universities Press, 1976.

Benson, H. The relaxation response. New York: Morrow, Inc., 1975.

Berkowitz, B., and Graziano, A. Training parents as behavior therapists: A review. Behav Res Ther, 1972, 10, 297-317.

Bowers, K. S., and Kelly, P. Stress, disease, psychotherapy, and hypnosis. J Abnorm Psychol, 1979, 88, 490-505.

Chandler, L. A. What teachers can do about childhood stress. Phi Delta Kappan, Dec., 1981, 63, 276-278.

Chandler, L. A. Brief therapy: Ronny G. Psychology in the Schools, 1983, 20, 215-218.

Clarizio, H. F., and McCoy, G. F. Behavior disorders of children. New York: Thomas Crowell Co., 1976.

Conners, C., Eisenberg, L., and Sharpe, L. A controlled study of the differential application of outpatient psychiatric treatment for children. Jpn J Child Psychiatry, 1965, 6, 125-132.

Conners, C., and Werry, J. Pharmacotherapy. In H. C. Quay and J. Werry (Eds.), Psychopathological disorders of childhood (2nd Ed.). New York: Wiley, 1979.

Critelli, J. W., and Neumann, K. F. The placebo: Conceptual analysis of a construct in transition. Am Psychol, 1984, 39, 32-39.

Day, R. C., and Sendak, S. N. The effect of Benson's relaxation response on the anxiety levels of Lebanese children under stress. J Exp Child Psychol, 1982, 34, 350-356.

Douglas, V. I. Stop, look and listen: The problem of sustained attention and impulse control in hyperactive and normal children. Can J Behav Sci, 1972, 4, 259-281.

Douglas, V. I., Parry, P., Marton, P., Assessment of a cognitive training p active children. J Abnorm Child Psy 389-410.

Eisenberg, L., Gilbert, A., Cytryn, L., an The effectiveness of psychotherapy alon junction with perphenazine or placebo i of neurotic and hyperkinetic children. 1961, 117, 1088-1093.

Fish, J. M. Placebo therapy: A practical gu influence in psychotherapy. San Francisc Jossey-Bass, 1973.

Frank, J. D. Persuasion and healing. Baltimor Hopkins Press, 1961.

Gaardner, K., and Montgomery, P. Clinical biofee A procedural manual. Baltimore: Williams an Wilkins Co., 1977.

Humphrey, J. N. Creative relaxation: A stress red technique for children. In J. H. Humphrey (Ed. Stress in childhood. New York: AMS Press, 1984

Jacobsen, F. Progressive relaxation. Chicago: Unive of Chicago Press, 1938.

Jacobsen, F. Variations of blood pressure with skeletal muscle tension and relaxation. Ann Intern Med, 193 16, 1619-1623.

Johnson, S. B. Anxiety in children: Recent advances in prevention. Paper presented at the annual meeting of the American Psychological Association, Washington, D.C., 1982.

Kipper, D. A., and Gilardi, D. Effectiveness of structured psychodrama and systematic desensitization in reducing test anxiety. J Counseling Psychol, 1978, 25, 499-505.

Lupin, M. N., Braud, L. W., Braud, W. G., and Duer, W. F. Children, parents and relaxation tapes. Academic Therapy, 1976, 12, 106-113.

Meichenbaum, D. A self-instructional approach to stress management: A proposal for stress inoculation training. In C. Spielberger and I. Sarason (Eds.), Stress and anxiety (Vol. 2). New York: Wiley, 1975.

Meichenbaum, D. Cognitive-behavioral modification: Future directions. In P. Sjoden et al. (Eds.), Trends in behavior therapy. New York: Academic Press, 1979.

Meichenbaum, D., and Asarnow, J. Cognitive-behavioral modification and metacognitive development: Implications for the classroom. In P. Kendall and S. Hollon (Eds.), Cognitive-behavioral interventions: Theory, research and procedures. New York: Academic Press, 1979.

Meichenbaum, D., and Goodman, J. Training impulsive children to talk to themselves: A means of developing self control. J Abnorm Psychol, 1971, 77, 115-126.

Miller, N. E. Learning of visceral and glandular responses. Science, 1969, 163, 434-445.

Miller, N. E. Biofeedback and visceral learning. Annu Rev Psychol, 1978, 29, 373-404.

Novaco, R. The cognitive regulation of anger and stress. In P. Kendall and S. Hollon (Eds.), Cognitive-behavioral interventions: Theory, research and procedures. New York: Academic Press, 1979.

Nuechterlein, K. H., and Holyrod, J. C. Biofeedback in the treatment of tension headache. Arch Gen Psychiatry, 1980, 37, 866-873.

Palkes, H., Stewart, M., and Kahana, B. Porteus Maze performance of hyperactive boys after training in self-directed verbal commands. Child Dev, 1968, 39, 817-829.

Patel, C. H. Yoga and biofeedback in the management of hypertension. In D. Wheatley (Ed.), Stress and the heart. New York: Raven Press, 1981.

Douglas, V. I., Parry, P., Marton, P., and Garson, C. Assessment of a cognitive training program for hyperactive children. J Abnorm Child Psychol, 1976, 4, 389-410.

Eisenberg, L., Gilbert, A., Cytryn, L., and Molling, P. The effectiveness of psychotherapy alone and in conjunction with perphenazine or placebo in the treatment of neurotic and hyperkinetic children. Am J Psychiatry, 1961, 117, 1088-1093.

Fish, J. M. Placebo therapy: A practical guide to social influence in psychotherapy. San Francisco, Calif.: Jossey-Bass, 1973.

Frank, J. D. Persuasion and healing. Baltimore: Johns Hopkins Press, 1961.

Gaardner, K., and Montgomery, P. Clinical biofeedback: A procedural manual. Baltimore: Williams and Wilkins Co., 1977.

Humphrey, J. N. Creative relaxation: A stress reduction technique for children. In J. H. Humphrey (Ed.), Stress in childhood. New York: AMS Press, 1984.

Jacobsen, F. Progressive relaxation. Chicago: University of Chicago Press, 1938.

Jacobsen, F. Variations of blood pressure with skeletal muscle tension and relaxation. Ann Intern Med, 1939, 16, 1619-1623.

Johnson, S. B. Anxiety in children: Recent advances in prevention. Paper presented at the annual meeting of the American Psychological Association, Washington, D.C., 1982.

Kipper, D. A., and Gilardi, D. Effectiveness of structured psychodrama and systematic desensitization in reducing test anxiety. J Counseling Psychol, 1978, 25, 499-505.

Lupin, M. N., Braud, L. W., Braud, W. G., and Duer, W. F. Children, parents and relaxation tapes. Academic Therapy, 1976, 12, 106-113.

Beck, A. T. Cognitive therapy and emotional disorders. New York: International Universities Press, 1976.

Benson, H. The relaxation response. New York: Morrow, Inc., 1975.

Berkowitz, B., and Graziano, A. Training parents as behavior therapists: A review. Behav Res Ther, 1972, 10, 297-317.

Bowers, K. S., and Kelly, P. Stress, disease, psychotherapy, and hypnosis. J Abnorm Psychol, 1979, 88, 490-505.

Chandler, L. A. What teachers can do about childhood stress. Phi Delta Kappan, Dec., 1981, 63, 276-278.

Chandler, L. A. Brief therapy: Ronny G. Psychology in the Schools, 1983, 20, 215-218.

Clarizio, H. F., and McCoy, G. F. Behavior disorders of children. New York: Thomas Crowell Co., 1976.

Conners, C., Eisenberg, L., and Sharpe, L. A controlled study of the differential application of outpatient psychiatric treatment for children. Jpn J Child Psychiatry, 1965, 6, 125-132.

Conners, C., and Werry, J. Pharmacotherapy. In H. C. Quay and J. Werry (Eds.), Psychopathological disorders of childhood (2nd Ed.). New York: Wiley, 1979.

Critelli, J. W., and Neumann, K. F. The placebo: Conceptual analysis of a construct in transition. Am Psychol, 1984, 39, 32-39.

Day, R. C., and Sendak, S. N. The effect of Benson's relaxation response on the anxiety levels of Lebanese children under stress. J Exp Child Psychol, 1982, 34, 350-356.

Douglas, V. I. Stop, look and listen: The problem of sustained attention and impulse control in hyperactive and normal children. Can J Behav Sci, 1972, 4, 259-281.

as sharing, along with such elements of the therapeutic relationship as the patient's faith and wish to trust, some responsibility for the efficacy of treatment. Suggestion and ritual are two elements of the placebo effect which, they maintain, have considerable potential within themselves.

Bowers and Kelly (1979) have provided evidence for the role of suggestion and hypnotic susceptibility in the psychological treatment of stress-related disorders. They argue that even in those interventions that are not explicitly hypnotic, suggestion and hypnotic susceptibility may be hidden factors that promote healing.

Their discussion of psychotherapy in relation to stress-induced disorders is worth reviewing here. Bowers and Kelly conceptualize the psychotherapeutic attempts to treat psychosomatic disorders along a continuum of specificity. Least specific are the conventional psychotherapies that have as their aim better psychological functioning. Next are those techniques that focus on reducing stress by lessening the threatening characteristics of the environment or increasing the patient's resources to cope more effectively. Finally, they consider the most specific therapies to be those that focus on ameliorating or eliminating some particular somatic dysfunction. They see biofeedback and relaxation techniques as being in this group. With those methods, and with many of the other techniques designed to assist in stress management, suggestion and the client's susceptibility to hypnosis seem to be common elements.

REFERENCES

Allen, K., and Harris, F. Elimination of a child's excessive scratching by training the mother in reinforcement procedures. Behav Res Ther, 1966, 4, 79-84.

Amar, P. B. Application of biofeedback training in children. In G. P. Sholevar et al. (Eds.), Emotional disorders in children and adolescents. New York: Spectrum, 1980.

Barten, H. H., and Barten, S. S. (Eds.). Children and their parents in brief therapy. New York: Behavioral Publications, 1973.

Paul, G. L. Physiological effects of relaxation training and hypnotic suggestion. J Abnorm Psychol, 1969, 74, 425-432.

Richardson, G. E., Beall, B. S., and Jessup, G. T. The effects of a high school stress management unit on student's heart rate and muscle tension. J School Health, 1982, 52, 229-233.

Rosenthal, A. J. Brief psychotherapy. In G. P. Sholevar et al. (Eds.), Emotional disorders in children and adolescents. New York: Spectrum, 1980.

Rosenthal, D., and Frank, J. D. Psychotherapy and the placebo effect. Psychol Bull, 1956, 53, 294-302.

Simpson, R., and Poplin, M. Parents as agents of change. Psychol Rev, 1981, 10, 15-25.

Stoyva, J., and Anderson, C. A coping-rest model of relaxation and stress management. In L. Goldberger and S. Breznitz (Eds.), Handbook of stress: Theoretical and clinical aspects. New York: The Free Press, 1982.

Stroebel, E. L., and Stroebel, C. F. The Quieting Reflex: A psychophysiologic approach for helping children deal with healthy and unhealthy stress. In J. H. Humphrey (Ed.), Stress in childhood. New York: AMS Press, 1984.

Suinn, R. M., and Deffenbacher, J. L. Behavior therapy. In I. L. Kutash et al. (Eds.), Handbook on stress and anxiety. San Francisco, Calif.: Jossey-Bass, 1980.

White, R., and Watt, N. The abnormal personality (4th Ed.). New York: Ronald Press, 1973.

Wolpe, J. Psychotherapy by reciprocal inhibition. Stanford, Calif.: Stanford University Press, 1958.

Wolpe, J. The practice of behavior therapy (3rd Ed.). New York: Pergamon Press, 1982.

APPENDIX

SAMPLE ONLY

PSYCHOLOGICAL ASSESSMENT

Name: Julie White	Date of Birth: January 22, 1977
Grade: Second	Date of Assessment: May 21, 1984
School: Lincoln Park	Age: 7 years, 4 months
District: Central	Examiner: S. Freud

Assessment Techniques and Results

Wechsler Intelligence Scale for Children--Revised
- Verbal IQ: 108
- Performance IQ: 114
- Full Scale IQ: 112

BASIS Achievement Test
- Reading Percentile Rank: 67
- Spelling Percentile Rank: 55
- Arithmetic Percentile Rank: 52

Stress Assessment System
- CLEI Percentile Rank: 06
- SRS Percentile Rank: 72
- Structured Parent Interview
- Children's Apperception Test

Reason for Referral

Julie is a seven-year-old second grader at the Lincoln Park School who has been referred for psychological assessment because of poor attentional skills and dependent behavior in the classroom. Her teachers describe her as a rather dependent child who often seeks approval and assurance from teachers and peers. They are concerned about what they regard as her excessive social behavior.

SAMPLE ONLY

PSYCHOLOGICAL ASSESSMENT

Name: David Green	Date of Birth: September 4, 1975
Grade: Fourth	Date of Assessment: June 6, 1984
School: Washington	Age: 8 years, 9 months
District: Union	Examiner: S. Freud

Assessment Techniques and Results

Wechsler Intelligence Scale for Children--Revised
- Verbal IQ: 98
- Performance IQ: 118
- Full Scale IQ: 108

BASIS Achievement Test
- Reading Percentile Rank: 28
- Spelling Percentile Rank: 32
- Arithmetic Percentile Rank: 22

Stress Assessment System
- CLEI Percentile Rank: 98
- SRS Percentile Rank: 92
- Structured Parent Interview
- Children's Apperception Test

Reason for Referral

David is an eight-year-old fourth grader at the Washington Elementary School who has been referred for psychological assessment because of poor school performance and behavior problems. He is reported to be about one year below academic expectations. Lately there have been increasing reports of behavior problems at school including: refusal to work, defiance of authority, destruction of property, and problems with peers.

Observations

David was initially defensive and resistant to testing. He had to be rather firmly reminded of the limits of the testing situation, but once these were made clear to him, he was able to work, and even showed some interest in the nonverbal tasks. As a result of his shifting adjustment to the situation, his motivation varied widely. At times he became oppositional, but this seemed to be more of a testing of limits than an absolute refusal since, when reminded that the work was inevitable, he acquiesced. David's behavioral style reflected some of the difficulties reported in social relations. He would alternate between polite acquiescence and open defiance in an attempt to manipulate the situation. When met with adult consistency, however, he was able to meet the demands of the situation.

Intellective Assessment

Assessment of David's intellectual ability suggests that he is functioning in the average range of intelligence. His Full Scale IQ score of 108 places him at the 70th percentile when compared to a normative sample of children at his same age level. The chances are 95 out of 100 that his true score will lie in the range from 102 to 114. These results suggest that David has the intellectual potential for at least average school work at his age/grade expectancy level.

Achievement Assessment

David's performance on the academic achievement test indicates that his overall academic level is somewhat below what might be expected for a child of his intellectual ability. David's reading score places him at the 28th percentile; his arithmetic score at the 22nd percentile; and his spelling score at the 32nd percentile. The pattern of the scores, along with the scores from the intelligence test, show no indication of a specific learning disability.

Stress Assessment

A review of his developmental history shows no reported health problems that might increase David's vulnerability to stress.

A survey of David's life history and current situation has identified 17 potentially stressful life events:

starting school, birth of brother, loss of job by parent, death of grandmother, mother beginning to work, changed schools, increase in arguments with siblings, academic failure, learning problems in school, frequent absence of parent, suspension from school, divorce of parents, family moves and relocations, poor grades in school, marriage of parent to step-parent, marital separation, and increase in number of arguments with parent. Subsequent interviews revealed that David's parents had been divorced when he was two years old, and he lived with his mother until recently. There are indications that his life with her was unstable and erratic; recently his father has assumed custody. The considerable number of potentially stressful life events means that when compared with a normative population of other eight-year-olds, David is placed at the 98th percentile, and at a high range of risk on this measure.

An analysis of significant needs and threats based on David's projective thematic responses suggests that his most frequent concerns have to do with aggression and being aggressed against by persons in his environment. There are also indications of fears of insecurity and rejection.

David tends to respond to stress situations by adopting an impulsive, acting-out behavioral style characterized by excited, restless, distracted, and overactive behavior with frequent fights and temper outbursts. Teacher ratings place his behavior at the level of a severe adjustment reaction.

An analysis of the effects of stress suggests that school, family, and social functioning are being affected. His school work has been affected to the point where it is unlikely that he will be able to meet the demands of the fifth grade without considerable intervention.

In summary, David's life stress assessment indicates that he is experiencing considerable stress due to a series of disruptive life events and environmental chaos. His unstable environment has caused him to adopt an impulsive, acting-out response style in reaction to stress.

Summary of Results

David is an eight-year-old fourth grader of average intelligence who is showing a number of behavior problems that are significantly interfering with his ability to work in school and to develop normal social relations. It appears that this behavior is in response to a series of stressful life events and an unstable, stressful environment.

SAMPLE ONLY

PSYCHOLOGICAL ASSESSMENT

Name: Karrie Brown	Date of Birth: December 4, 1974
Grade: Third	Date of Assessment: June 9, 1984
School: Greenwood	Age: 9 years, 6 months
District: Forest	Examiner: S. Freud

Assessment Techniques and Results

Wechsler Intelligence Scale for Children--Revised
- Verbal IQ: 110
- Performance IQ: 108
- Full Scale IQ: 111

BASIS Achievement Test
- Reading Percentile Rank: 77
- Spelling Percentile Rank: 82
- Arithmetic Percentile Rank: 74

Stress Assessment System
- CLEI Percentile Rank: 44
- SRS Percentile Rank: 55
- Structured Parent Interview
- Children's Apperception Test

Reason for Referral

Karrie is a nine-year-old third grader at the Greenwood Elementary School who has been referred for psychological assessment because her parents feel that she tends to daydream and procrastinate in getting her school work done. Her teachers report that her grades have been average, and they see no evidence of learning problems.

Observations

Karrie was tentative and reticent in her responses in the test situation. She generally appeared quiet and reserved, and made no spontaneous comments. Karrie seemed uncertain about her capabilities. For example, she was unwilling to guess when in doubt, couched her responses in self-critical statements, and frequently erased her answers. As the tasks increased in difficulty, her tolerance for frustration diminished markedly.

Intellective Assessment

Assessment of Karrie's intellectual ability suggests that she is functioning in the above average range of intelligence. Her Full Scale IQ score of 111 places her at the 77th percentile when compared to a normative sample of children at her same age level. The chances are 95 out of 100 that her true score will lie in the range from 105 to 117. These results suggest that Karrie has the intellectual potential for schoolwork at or somewhat above her age/grade expectancy level.

Achievement Assessment

Karrie's performance on the academic achievement test indicates that her overall academic level is near to that which might be expected for a child of her intellectual ability. Karrie's reading score places her at the 77th percentile; her arithmetic score at the 74th percentile; and her spelling score at the 82nd percentile. The pattern of scores, along with the scores from the intelligence test, shows no indication of a specific learning disability.

Stress Assessment

A review of her developmental history shows no reported health problems that might increase Karrie's vulnerability to stress.

A survey of Karrie's life history and current situation has identified five potentially stressful life events: beginning school, mother starting to work, death of grandparent, family moves and relocations, and frequent absence of one or both parents.

An analysis of significant needs and threats based on Karrie's thematic responses suggests there is considerable concern over needs for affiliation and achievement.

Thematic analysis showed strong needs for nurturance, support, and family belonging. Perceived parental demands for achievement are also a source of considerable stress for Karrie.

Karrie tends to respond to stress by occasionally adopting extreme behaviors. She tends to be playful and easily distracted, and she seldom completes tasks.

An analysis of the effects of stress suggests that there are some somatic symptoms that might be associated with a stress reaction, that is, mild occurrences of allergies and asthma. While there seems to have been little impact on family and social functioning, schoolwork may be somewhat impaired. The effects of stress may be seen in her problems with attention, concentration, and memory.

In summary, Karrie's life stress assessment indicates that she is a nine-year-old with normal developmental needs and some slight adjustment difficulties precipitated by specific environmental stressors, that is, frequent moves and relocations and the intermittent availability of her parents. As a result, she feels that her needs for nurturance are not being adequately met. In addition, because she has associated family support with continued achievement, problems in school functioning are particularly stressful for Karrie.

Summary of Results

Karrie is a nine-year-old of above average intelligence who is showing some difficulties in functioning in school. These difficulties may be associated with a series of environmental stressors in her recent past with which she appears to have had at least some partial success in coping.

SAMPLE ONLY

PSYCHOLOGICAL ASSESSMENT

Name: Jeremy Jones	Date of Birth: January 15, 1977
Grade: First	Date of Assessment: June 23, 1984
School: Greendale	Age: 7 years, 5 months
District: Green Valley	Examiner: S. Freud

Assessment Techniques and Results

Wechsler Intelligence Scale for Children--Revised
Verbal IQ: 96
Performance IQ: 106
Full Scale IQ: 101

BASIS Achievement Test
Reading Percentile Rank: 32
Arithmetic Percentile Rank: 27
Spelling Percentile Rank: 30

Stress Assessment System
CLEI Percentile Rank: 55
SRS Percentile Rank: 57
Structured Parent Interview
Children's Apperception Test

Reason for Referral

Jeremy is a seven-year-old first grader at the Greendale Elementary School who has been referred for psychological assessment because of his declining school performance. He is reported to be working below his peers in most academic areas, especially in reading, for which he receives remedial instruction. His teacher is recommending that he be retained in the first grade.

Observations

Jeremy was somewhat reluctant, but after some encouragement, he willingly accompanied the examiner. Jeremy's behavior during the testing was cooperative, although his behavior suggested that his social awareness and maturity is somewhat underdeveloped. Jeremy's approaches to the verbal and nonverbal tasks varied widely. While he frequently yawned and commented that he was tired during the verbal tasks, he eagerly attempted to solve the nonverbal problems, often exclaiming, "This is fun!" Although he did not appear to be overly concerned with his performance, he stated that he hoped that his father would be pleased with his test score.

Intellective Assessment

Assessment of Jeremy's intellectual ability suggests that he is functioning in the average range of intelligence. His Full Scale IQ score of 101 places him at the 53rd percentile when compared to a normative sample of children at his same age level. The chances are 95 out of 100 that his true score will lie in the range from 94 to 108. These results suggest that a lack of intellectual ability may be ruled out as a probable cause for his poor school performance.

Achievement Assessment

Jeremy's performance on the academic achievement test indicates that his overall academic level is somewhat below that expected for a child of his age. Jeremy's reading score places him at the 32nd percentile; his arithmetic score at the 27th percentile; and his spelling score at the 30th percentile. When compared to a normative sample of children of his same age, his pattern of scores, along with the scores of the intelligence test, suggest that a specific learning disability may be ruled out as a probable cause of his poor school performance.

Stress Assessment

A review of his developmental history shows no reported health problems that might increase Jeremy's vulnerability to stress.

A review of Jeremy's history and current life situation has identified the following potentially stressful life events: academic failure, addition of a third party to the family, illness of sister requiring hospitalization, learning problems in school, speech problems, beginning school, family moving, and poor grades in school. This is a total of eight events which, when compared with a normative population of other seven-year-olds, places Jeremy at the 55th percentile, and at an average range of risk on this measure.

An analysis of significant needs and threats based on Jeremy's projective thematic responses suggests that his strongest concerns involve his needs for security and the concomitant threat of insecurity. In addition, there is evidence to suggest a particular sensitivity toward aggression/ punishment and achievement/failure situations.

Jeremy tends to respond to stress situations by adopting an impulsive behavioral style characterized by restlessness, overactivity, and nervous behavior. Parental ratings place his behavior at the level of a mild adjustment reaction.

An analysis of the effects of stress suggests that, while there has been relatively little impact on Jeremy's health, family, and social functioning, there has been considerable impact on his school functioning. Jeremy has shown difficulty in attending to school work, and problems in remembering material learned in school.

In summary, Jeremy's life stress assessment shows that significant sources of stress are found for him in those situations that might exacerbate his fears of failure, punishment, and insecurity. Jeremy is likely to respond impulsively in such stress situations. His impulsive, overactive responses impair his ability to attend and so increase the probability of further learning problems, thus creating additional stressors for Jeremy.

Summary of Results

Jeremy is a seven-year-old first grader of average intelligence who is showing problems in school functioning. There are no indications of a significant learning disability. Rather, it appears that Jeremy's problems may be the result of a reaction to perceived stress associated with threats of failure and insecurity.

SAMPLE ONLY

PSYCHOLOGICAL ASSESSMENT

Name: David Black
Grade: First
School: St. Joseph's
District: Western

Date of Birth: July 10, 1977
Date of Assessment: May 12, 1984
Age: 6 years, 10 months
Examiner: S. Freud

Assessment Techniques and Results

Wechsler Intelligence Scale for Children--Revised
- Verbal IQ: 199
- Performance IQ: 114
- Full Scale IQ: 119

BASIS Achievement Test
- Reading Percentile Rank: 62
- Spelling Percentile Rank: 74
- Arithmetic Percentile Rank: 48

Stress Assessment System
- CLEI Percentile Rank: 33
- SRS Percentile Rank: 65
- Structured Parent Interview
- Children's Apperception Test

Reason for Referral

David is a six-year-old first grader at St. Joseph's School who has been referred for psychological assessment because ne seems to be having problems in coping with schoolwork. His teachers describe him as a child who has a great difficulty completing his work. He occasionally daydreams, and shows frequent immature behavior in the classroom.

Observations

Initially, David adjusted well to the testing situation, and readily completed the required tasks. However, as the session progressed, he became increasingly restless, frequently inquiring when he would be finished. His increased restlessness did not seem to inhibit his ability to attend, although he did have to be reminded on occasion. For the most part David tended to respond impulsively, without careful reflection.

Intellective Assessment

Assessment of David's intellectual ability suggests that he is functioning in the above average range of intelligence. His Full Scale IQ score of 119 places him at the 90th percentile when compared to a normative sample of children at his same age level. The chances are 95 out of 100 that his true score will lie in the range from 112 to 126. These results suggest that David has the intellectual potential necessary for schoolwork at or somewhat above his age/grade expectancy level.

Achievement Assessment

David's performance on the academic achievement test indicates that his overall academic level is slightly below what might be expected of a child with his intellectual ability. David's reading score places him at the 62nd percentile; his arithmetic score at the 48th percentile; and his spelling score at the 74th percentile. The pattern of scores, along with the scores from the intelligence test, show no indication of a specific learning disability.

Stress Assessment

A review of his developmental history shows no reported health problems that might increase David's vulnerability to stress.

A survey of David's life history and current situation has identified three potentially stressful life events: beginning school, learning problems, and a severe accident resulting in the hospitalization of his sister. The latter occurred when there was a fire in the home when David was two years old. Although he escaped unharmed, his sister was severely burned, and subsequently an inordinate amount of parental time was spent taking her for frequent treatment at the burn clinic.

An analysis of significant needs and threats based on David's projective thematic responses suggests that there is considerable concern over the threat of insecurity, and the loss of independence. Thematic analysis shows specific concerns with physical danger, especially from fire, and a strong need to resist what is perceived as adult domination.

David tends to adopt a dependent response to stress characterized by playful, demanding, stubborn, and generally immature behavior. There are also indications of impulsive qualities in his behavioral pattern. Teacher ratings place his behavior at the level of a mild adjustment reaction.

An analysis of the effects of stress suggests that, for the most part, there have been relatively little physical effects, except for a problem with bedwetting, which has been of some duration. There are some indications of an impact on social relations, that is, David's use of his "helplessness" to manipulate others. There is also increasing evidence of an impact on school functioning. David seems to show little concern with completing school assignments, and generally seems unwilling to perform tasks that require independence and self-initiative to complete.

In summary, David's life stress assessment shows that there are three major sources of stress for him: (1) his fears of physical harm and the loss of parental protection which he associates with it. (2) The dependent style he tends to adopt in response to stress, while partially successful in allowing him to regress to a less demanding state, has created further problems by increasing the ambivalence he feels toward his emerging drive for independence. As a result, as David becomes more extreme in his dependency, his resentment grows along with his fears of losing independence. (3) The dependent response style has inhibited his initiative in school, and his childish resistance to domination has kept him from completing school assignments. The result is that he is now experiencing academic difficulties that are creating an additional source of stress.

Summary of Results

David is a six-year-old first grader of above average intelligence who is showing problems in school functioning. It appears that these problems are the result of real and perceived stressors in David's life experience, and his unsuccessful efforts to cope with them.

BIBLIOGRAPHY

The Children's Life Events Inventory

Chandler, L. A. (1981). The source of stress inventory. Psychology in the Schools, 18, 164-168.

Hoesch, A. H. (1982). Stressful life events of normal and clinic-referred children. Unpublished master's thesis, University of Pittsburgh.

Hoesch, A. H., and Chandler, L. A. (March, 1983). Stressful life events of children: Implications for screening and assessment. Paper presented at the convention of the National Association of School Psychologists, Detroit, Mich.

Hoesch, A. H. (1984). Stressful life events of children: Their frequency, magnitude, and classification. Unpublished doctoral dissertation, University of Pittsburgh.

Chandler, L. A. (1984). The Children's Life Events Inventory: Its use in clinical assessment. Unpublished paper, University of Pittsburgh.

Million, M. E. (1984). Stressful life events of children: Their relationship to socioeconomic status. Unpublished master's thesis, University of Pittsburgh.

Shermis, M. D., and Chandler, L. A. (1984). Scoring a children's life events inventory: Weighted versus unweighted scores. Unpublished paper, University of Pittsburgh.

Chandler, L. A., Million, M. E., and Shermis, M. D. (in press). The incidence of stressful life events of elementary school-aged children. American Journal of Community Psychology.

Chandler, L. A. (1985). The Children's Life Events Inventory: Validity and Reliability. Unpublished paper, University of Pittsburgh.

The Need-Threat Scoring System

Hughes, C. A. (1980). The reliability of a need-threat scoring system for projective material. Unpublished master's thesis, University of Pittsburgh.

Johnson, V. (1984). The use of a need-threat analysis of the Children's Apperception Test to discriminate between clinic-referred and nonreferred children. Unpublished master's thesis, University of Pittsburgh.

Chandler, L. A. (1984). Scoring the Children's Apperception Test using a need-threat analysis. Unpublished paper, University of Pittsburgh.

Chandler, L. A., and Hughes, C. A. (1984). The reliability of a need-threat scoring system for the Children's Apperception Test. Unpublished paper, University of Pittsburgh.

The Structured Parent Interview

Dubus, J. T. (1984). Obtaining baseline data on children using a structured parent interview. Unpublished master's thesis, University of Pittsburgh.

The Stress Response Scale

Chandler, L. A. (1979). A classification scheme for behavior disorders. Unpublished paper, University of Pittsburgh.

Piso, C. N. (1981). A revision, factor analysis, and concurrent validity study of a children's behavior scale. Unpublished doctoral dissertation, University of Pittsburgh.

Krotec, S. K. (1982). _A comparison of behavior, personality, and academic variables of learning disabled, emotionally disturbed, and normal adolescents._ Unpublished doctoral dissertation, University of Pittsburgh.

Chandler, L. A. (August, 1982). _The Stress Response Scale: A preliminary report._ Paper presented at the convention of the American Psychological Association, Washington, D.C.

Chandler, L. A., and Lundahl, W. T. (1983). Empirical classification of emotional adjustment reactions. _Am J Orthopsychiatry_, _53_, 460-467.

Chandler, L. A. (1983). The Stress Response Scale: An instrument for use in assessing emotional adjustment reactions. _School Psychol Rev_, _12_, 260-265.

Chandler, L. A. (1983). _The Stress Response Scale: A manual._ Unpublished paper, University of Pittsburgh.

Chandler, L. A. (1984). Behavioral responses of children to stress. In J. H. Humphrey (Ed.), _Stress in childhood._ New York: AMS Press, Inc.

Marsh, J. (1984). _An investigation into the validity and clinical use of the Stress Response Scale._ Unpublished master's project, University of Pittsburgh.

Chandler, L. A., Shermis, M. D., and Marsh, J. (1985). The use of the Stress Response Scale in diagnostic assessment. _J Psychoeducational Assess_, _3_ (1).

Robinson, M. (1985). _Predicting school psychologist's recommendations from ratings on the Stress Response Scale._ Unpublished doctoral dissertation, University of Pittsburgh.

Chandler, L. A., and Shermis, M. D. (in press). Assessing behavioral responses to stress. _Educational and Psychological Measurement._

System and System-Related

Siegel, D. J. (1981). Separation-loss events, self-concept, locus of control, and children's effective functioning in school. Unpublished doctoral dissertation, University of Pittsburgh.

Chandler, L. A. (December, 1981). What teachers can do about childhood stress. Phi Delta Kappan, 276-277.

Chandler, L. A. (1982). Children under stress: Understanding emotional adjustment reactions. Springfield, Ill.: Charles Thomas, Pub.

Chandler, L. A. (March, 1982). The Stress Assessment System: Assessing emotional adjustment reactions. Paper presented at the convention of the National Association of School Psychologists, Toronto, Canada.

Chandler, L. A., Hoesch, A. H., Hughes, C. A., and March, J. (April, 1984). The Stress Assessment System: Preliminary findings. Symposium presented at the convention of the National Association of School Psychologists, Philadelphia, Pa.

Kemmerer, A. (1984). A comparison of Stress Assessment System data of clinic-referred and non-referred children. Unpublished master's project, University of Pittsburgh.

Chandler, L. A. (in press). Towards a stress assessment system for children: A review of progress. In J. H. Humphrey (Ed.), Current selected research in stress. Princeton, N.J.: Princeton Book Co.

INDEX

academic performance (see school performance)
acting out, 6, 143
adaptation, 37, 38, 39, 47, 84, 100, 108, 113, 126, 130
adjustment, 2, 3, 4-6, 47, 49, 83-84, 90, 100, 105, 106, 108, 110, 113, 126, 127, 130, 132, 138, 147, 185
adolescence, 56-59, 84, 87, 106-7
aggression, 6, 88
anorexia nervosa, 78-80
anxiety, 36, 108, 109, 110, 186, 193, 194, 195, 197, 198
appraisal (see cognitive appraisal)
assessment, 3, 12-28, 147, 156, 160-63, 187
asthma, 74-76

Behavior disorders, 3, 17-18, 126, 130, 138, 143
biofeedback, 39, 191, 192-93, 198

Children's Apperception Test, 152-55
Children's Life Events Inventory, 147-52
cognitive appraisal, 37-38, 49, 100-101, 104-5, 128, 129
competence, 107-9, 114-15, 118-19, 126, 129
coping, 38, 59, 83, 86, 88, 116, 126, 127-30, 132, 136-38, 184, 186, 195-96; definition, 127
counseling, 186-90

death, 83, 84-86
dependent behavior, 85, 133-36, 142
depression, 6, 108, 118, 119, 130
desensitization, 193-94
disaster, 36, 40-42, 84, 102
disease, 38, 46, 112, 117-18
divorce, 5-6, 40, 45, 49, 83, 84, 86-89

ego strength, 100-105
emotional disorders, 2-3, 6-8, 13-18, 52, 77-78, 102, 112-13, 132, 138-40, 143
enuresis, 76-78

family, 41, 59, 77, 79-80, 83, 86, 101, 117, 126

gastrointestinal ulceration, 80-82, 117

hospitalization, 90, 107

illness, 38-43, 46, 101, 158
impulsive behavior, 6, 54, 136, 141-43

learning problems, 1
life events (see stress events)

need-threat scoring system, 152-55
needs, 36, 39, 50-51, 152-55

parental attitudes, 59, 87
parents, 2, 40-41, 59-60, 83, 84-86, 90, 102, 110, 116, 118, 126, 158, 185, 190
passive-aggressive behavior, 136, 141
perceived stress (see stress)
placebo, 197-99
problem-solving, 100, 109, 119, 126, 127, 196
projective techniques, 21-22, 152-55
psychoanalytic theory, 36, 79, 81, 116, 127, 186, 190
psychodynamic theory, 107, 117
psychophysiological reactions, 35, 37, 70-73, 158
psychosocial effects, 37, 38, 82-91
psychosomatic effects, 72-82, 159

relaxation, 39, 190-193, 195
repressed behavior, 136, 142

school performance, 1, 49, 55-56, 82, 85, 88-89, 118, 126
self-esteem, 105-6, 111, 115
special education, 2, 6-9
stress: definition of, 39; impact of, 1, 70-91, 126, 159; perceived situations of, 3, 39, 49-50, 53, 101, 104-5, 152-53; perceived situations of, 3, 39, 49-50, 53, 101, 104-5, 152-53
stress events, 40-51, 85, 100-101, 102, 147-52
stressors, 3; developmental, 51-59; social, 5, 59-61
Stress Response Scale, 140-43, 155-58
Structured Parent Interview, 158-60

teachers, 2, 4, 83, 126, 184, 185-86
temperament, 100, 102, 116, 138
threat, 36, 38, 39, 53, 71, 101, 104-5, 152-55
trauma, 3, 35-36, 37, 38, 40-42, 107, 110

ulcers (see gastrointestinal ulceration)

withdrawal, 1, 88

ABOUT THE AUTHOR

LOUIS A. CHANDLER, PH.D., received his undergraduate degree from Duquesne University, and has done graduate work there, at the New School for Social Research, and at the University of Pittsburgh. A former staff psychologist with the Exceptional Children's Program of the Allegheny Intermediate Unit, he has also served as a consulting psychologist to various community agencies and school districts. He is currently Clinical Associate Professor in the Department of Educational Psychology at the University of Pittsburgh, and Director of the University's Psychoeducational Clinic. Dr. Chandler is the author of numerous papers and articles on child psychology and of Children Under Stress, a practical guide for teachers and other professionals concerned with helping children. He is a member of the American Psychological Association, and the National Association of School Psychologists.